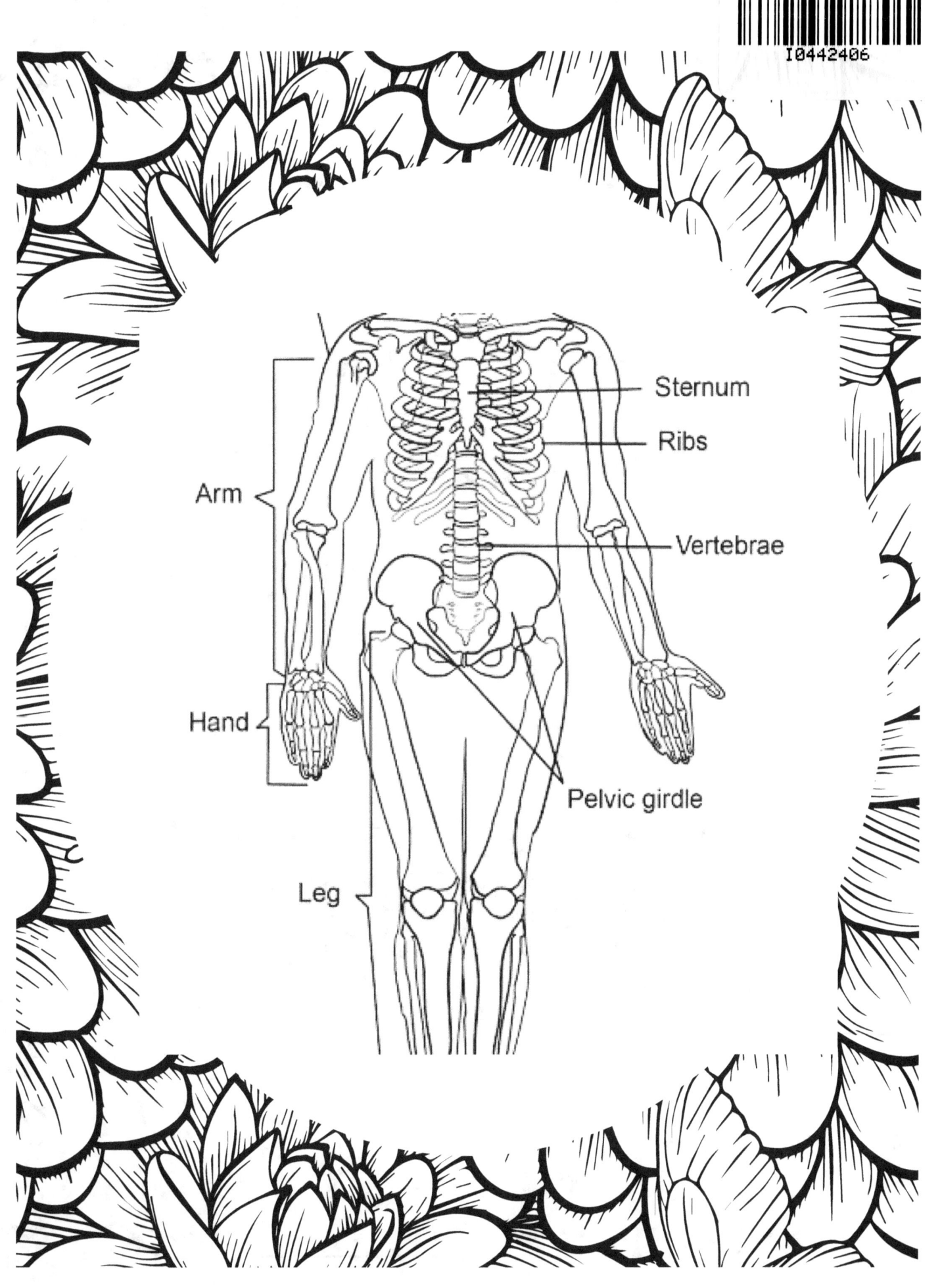

This Book Belongs To

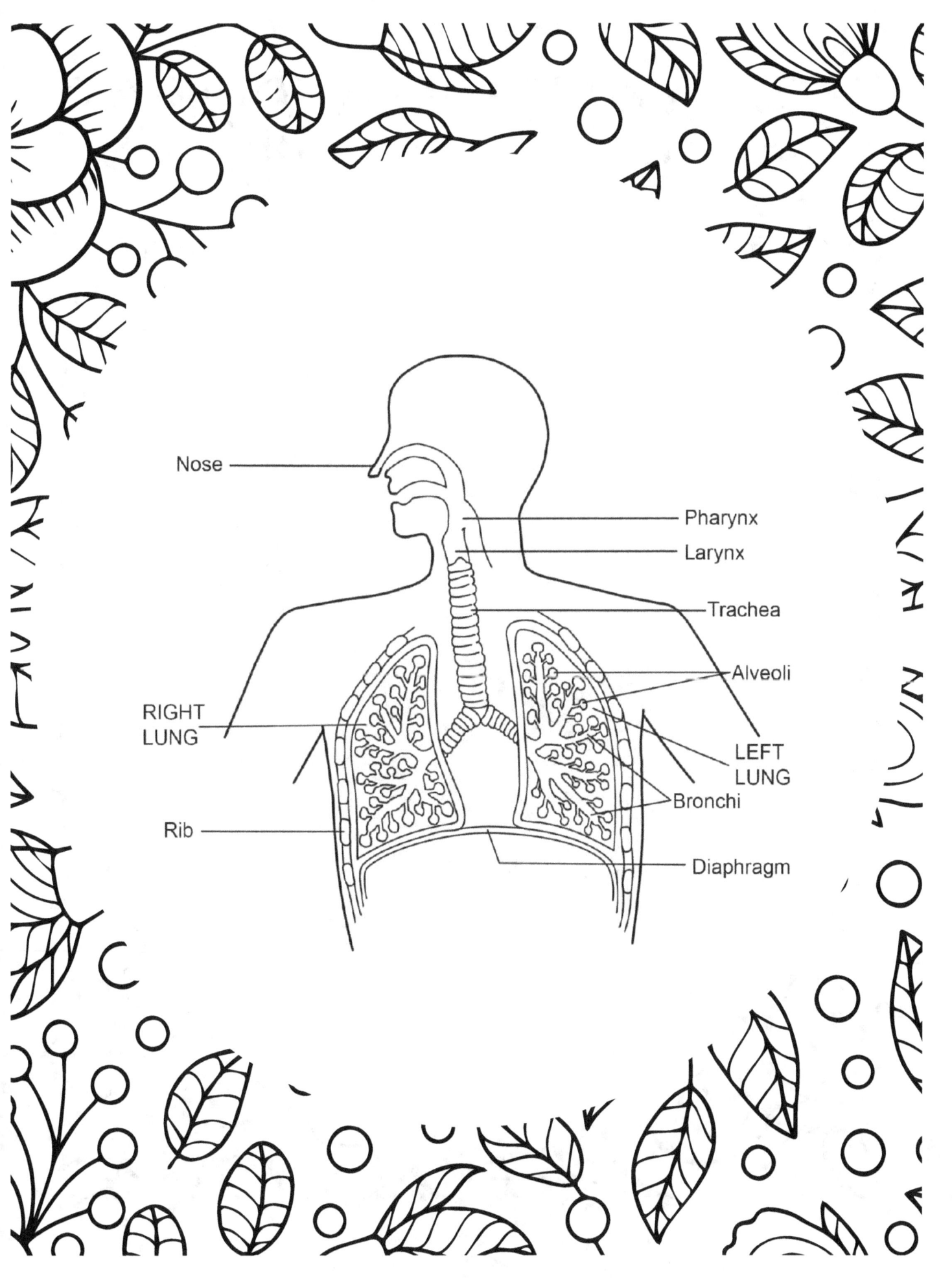

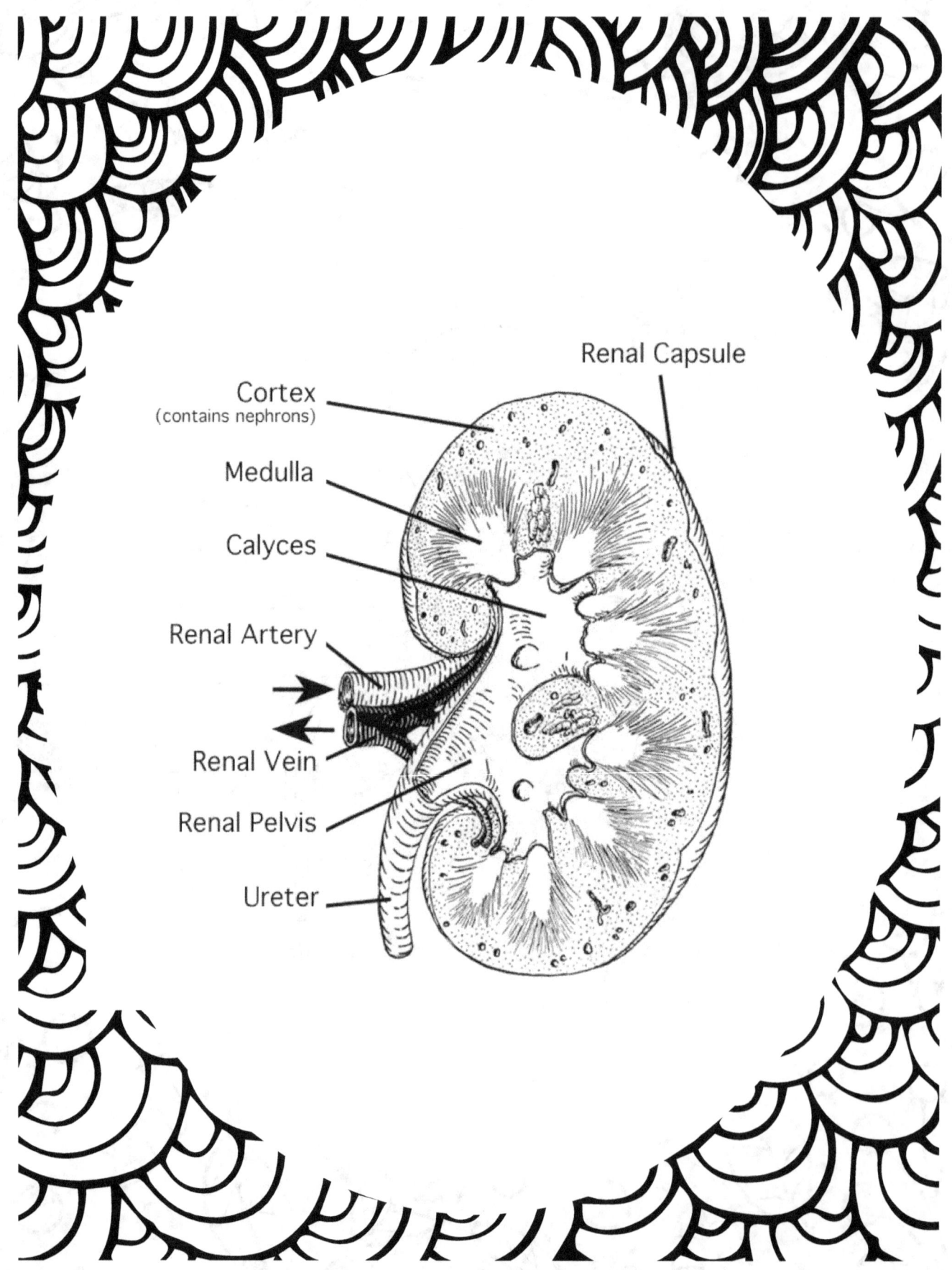

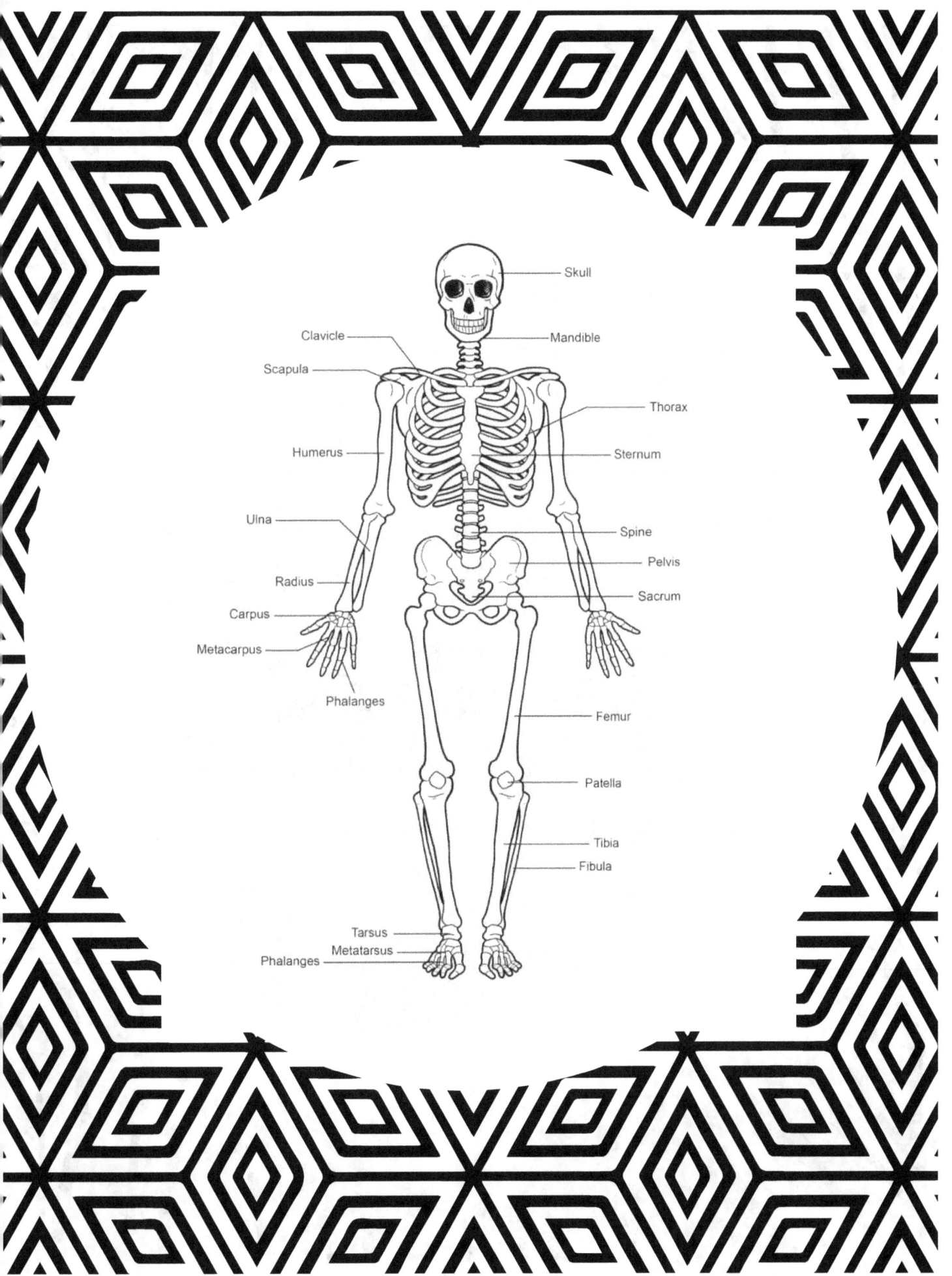

Color the Anatomy of the Knee Joint

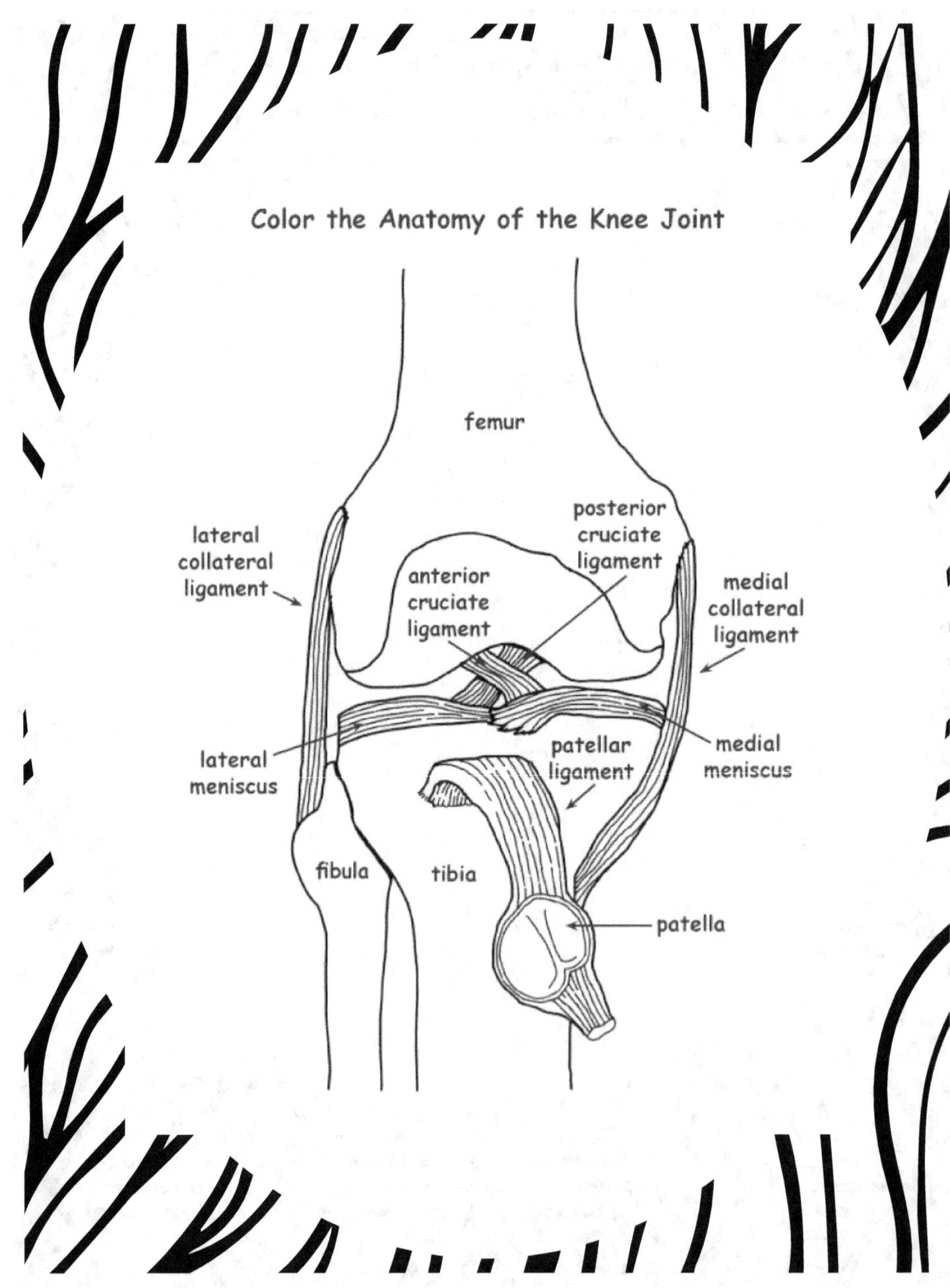

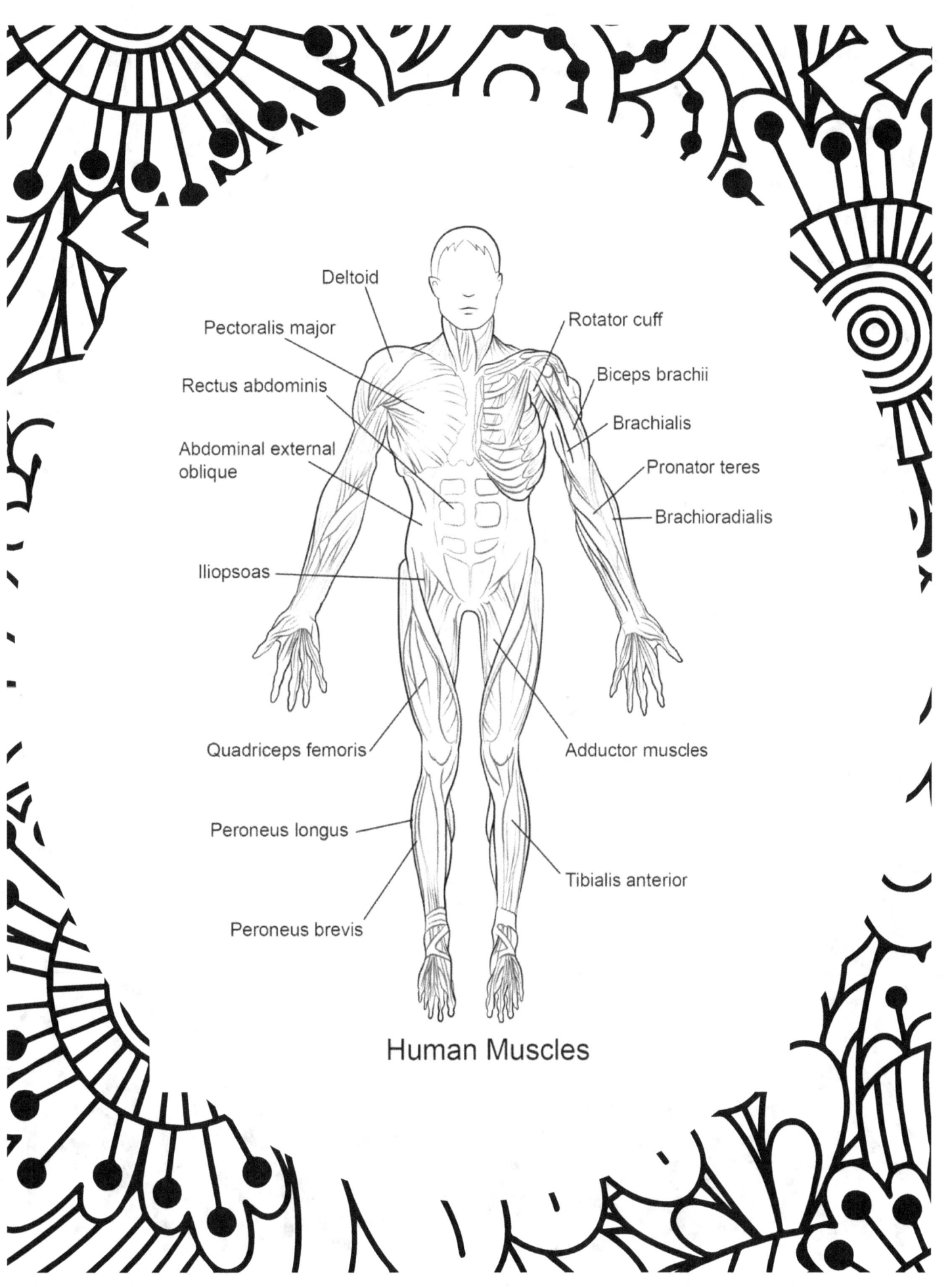

Human Muscles

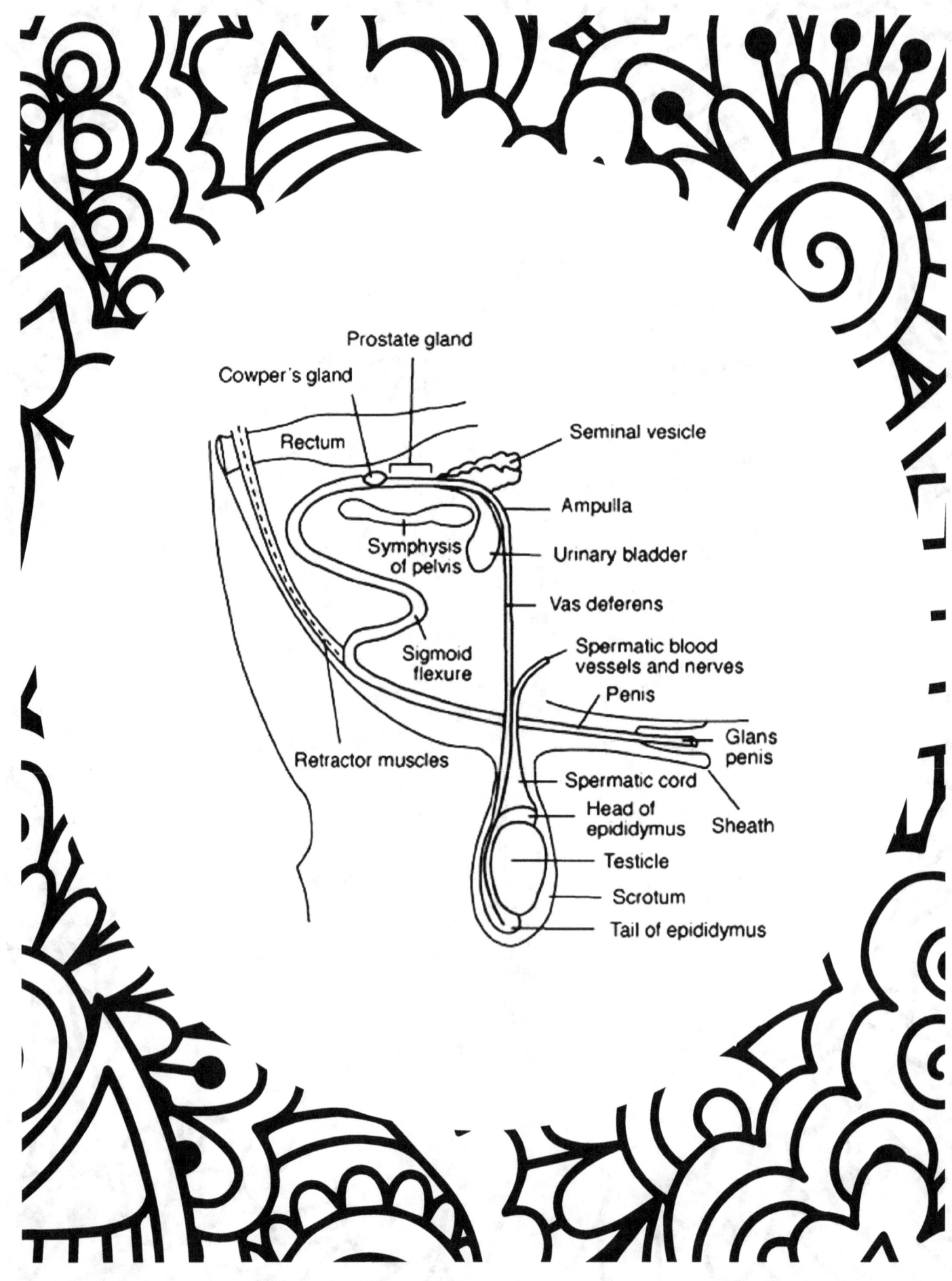

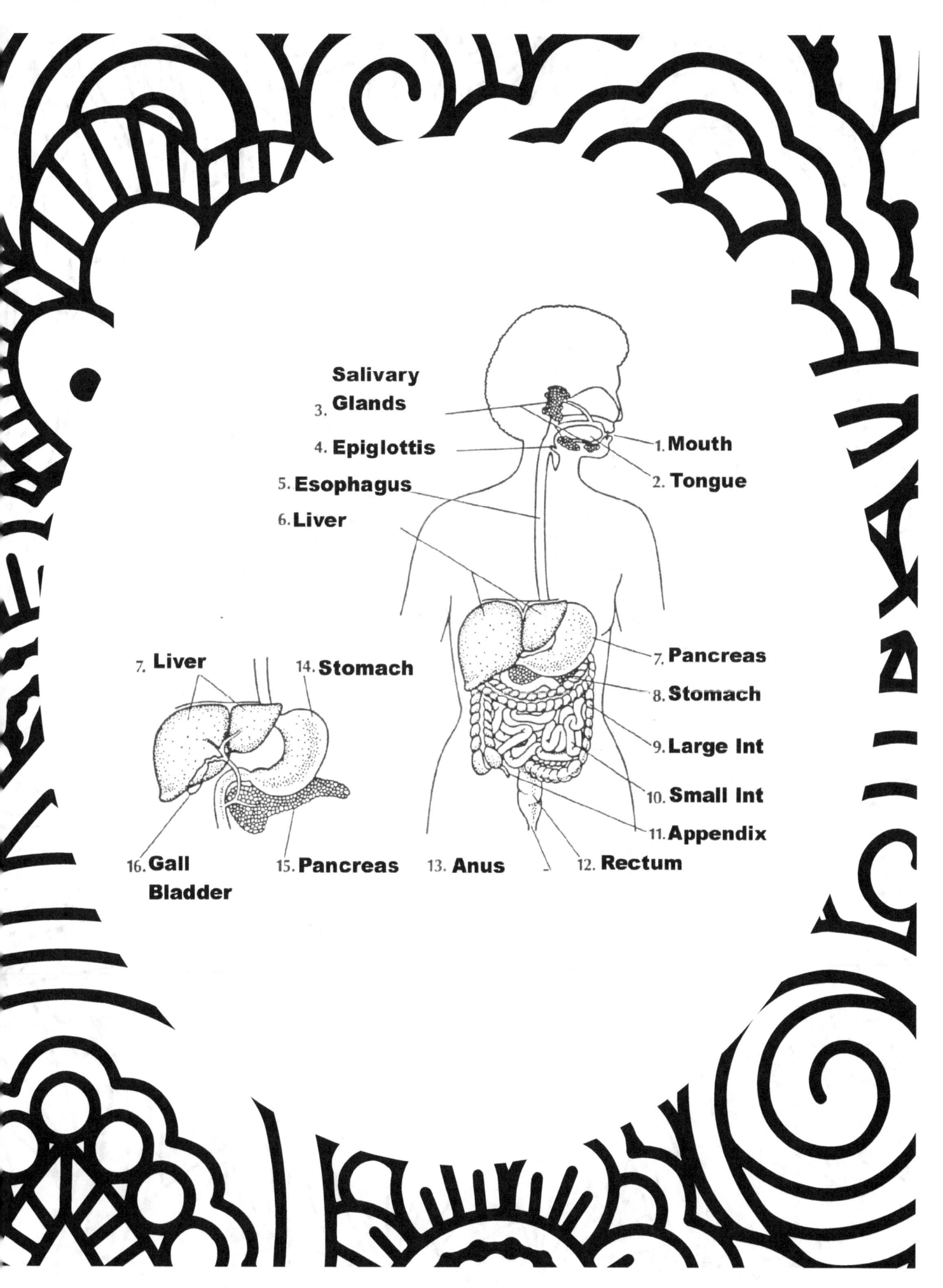

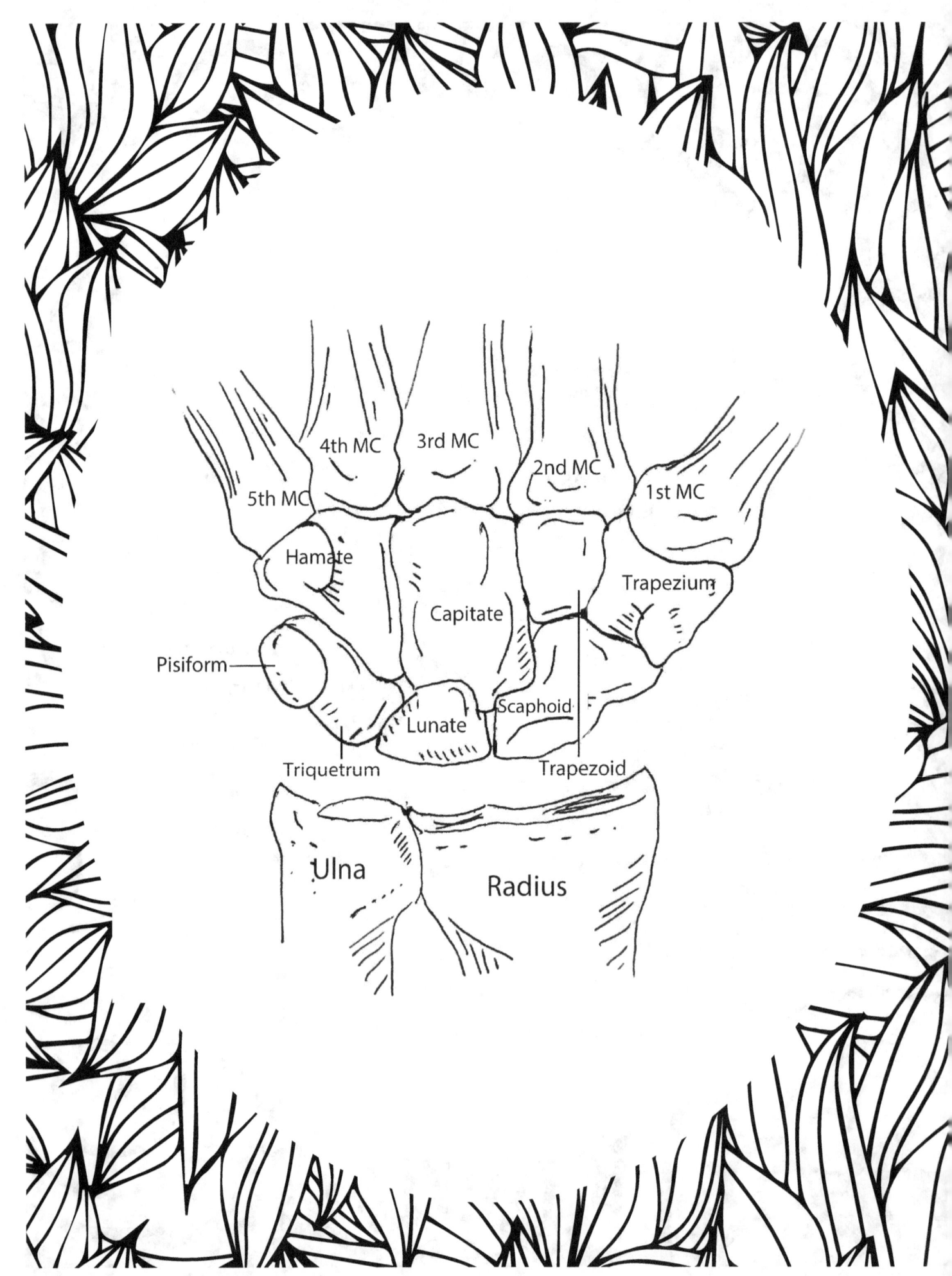

Color the Arteries of the Head and Neck

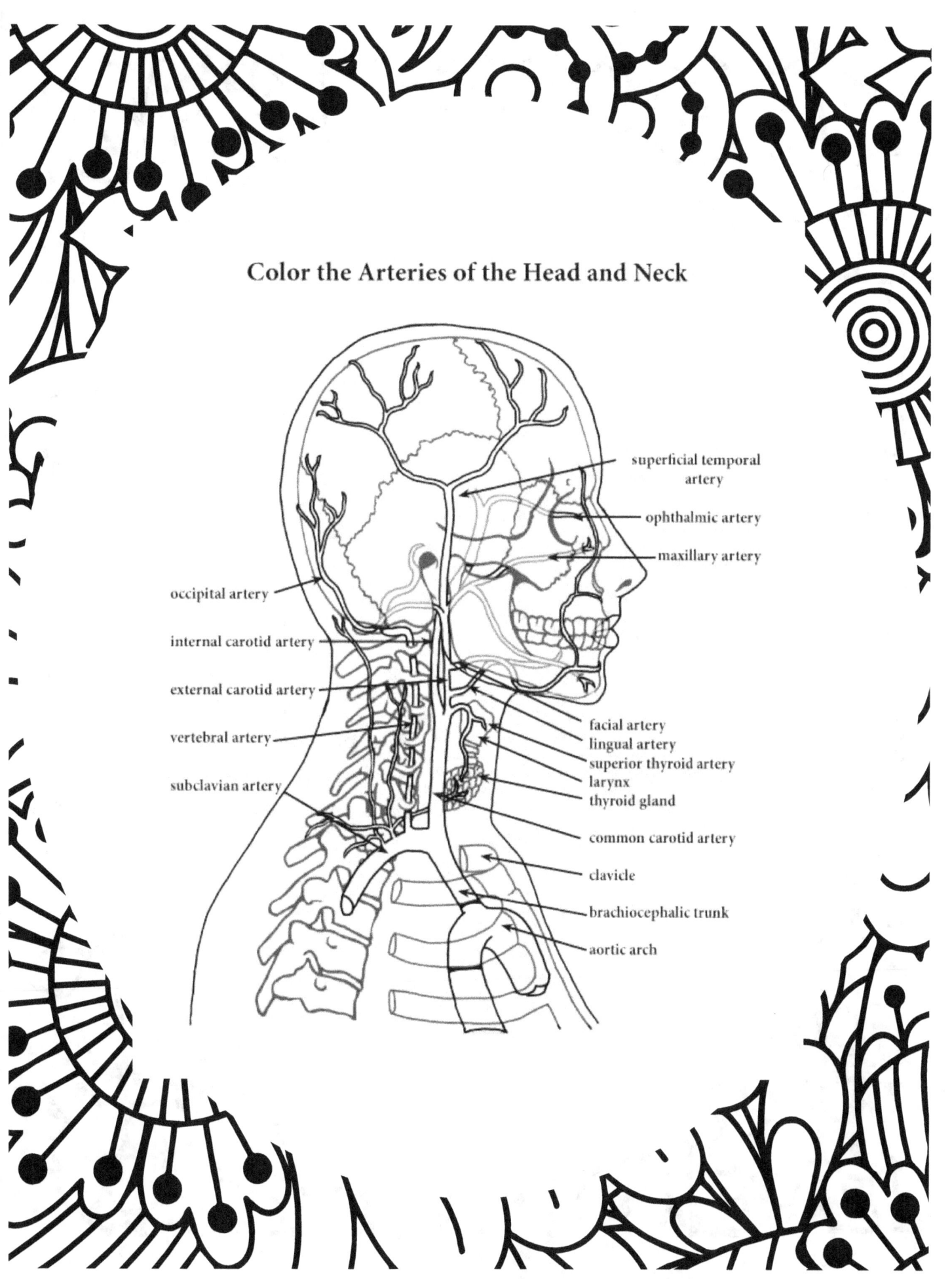

superficial temporal artery

ophthalmic artery

maxillary artery

occipital artery

internal carotid artery

external carotid artery

vertebral artery

subclavian artery

facial artery
lingual artery
superior thyroid artery
larynx
thyroid gland

common carotid artery

clavicle

brachiocephalic trunk

aortic arch

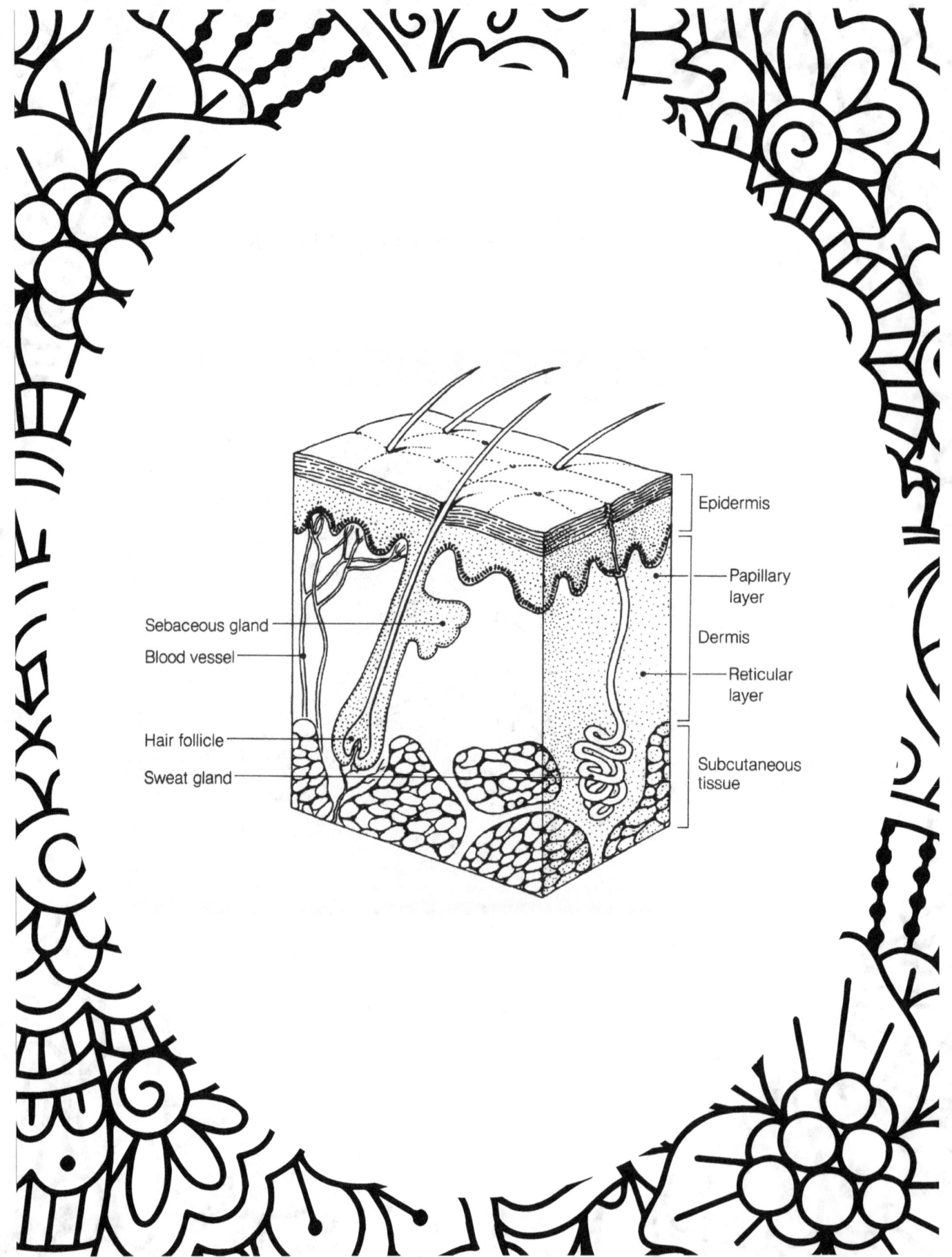

Epidermis

Papillary layer

Dermis

Reticular layer

Sebaceous gland

Blood vessel

Hair follicle

Sweat gland

Subcutaneous tissue

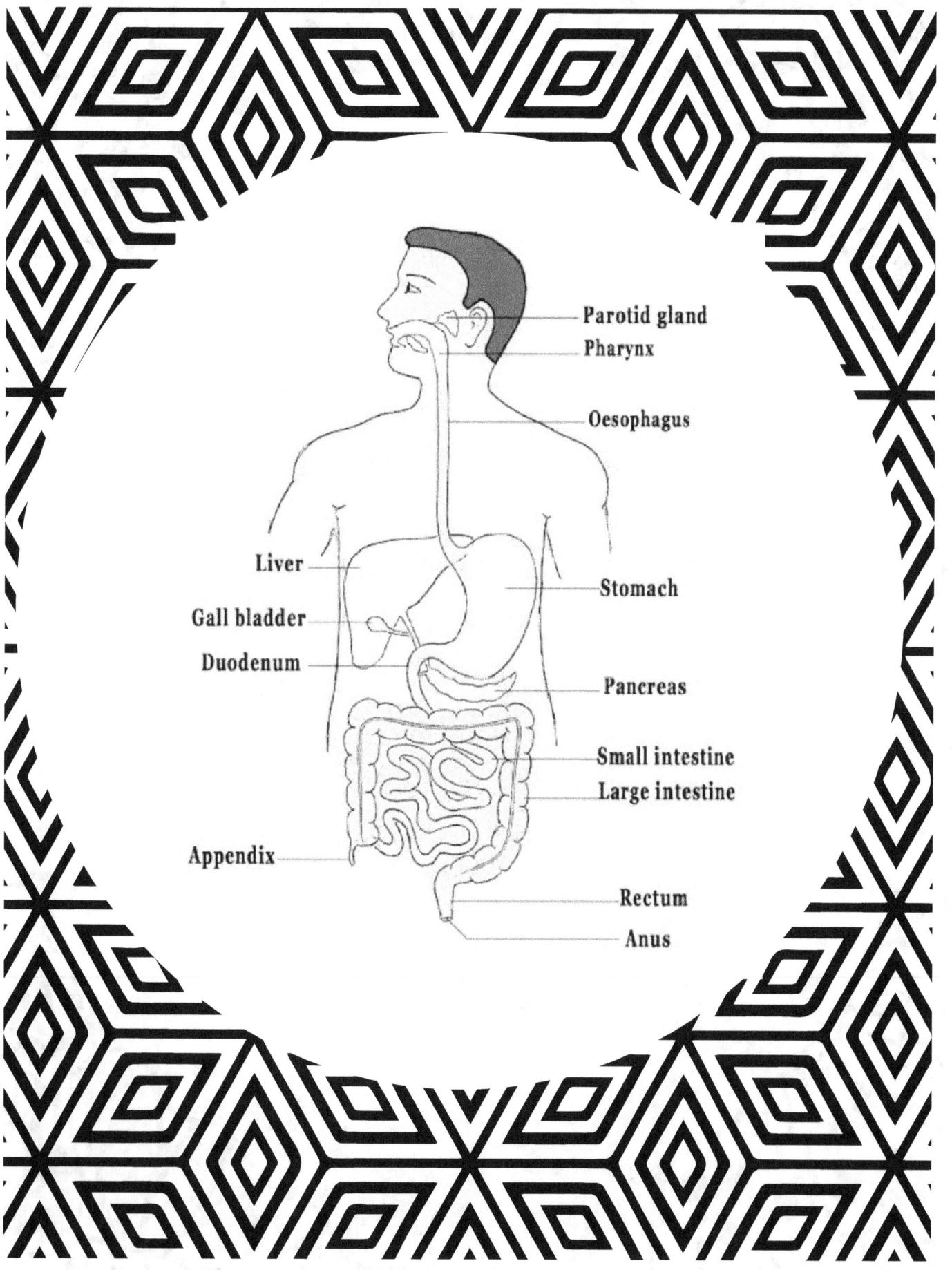

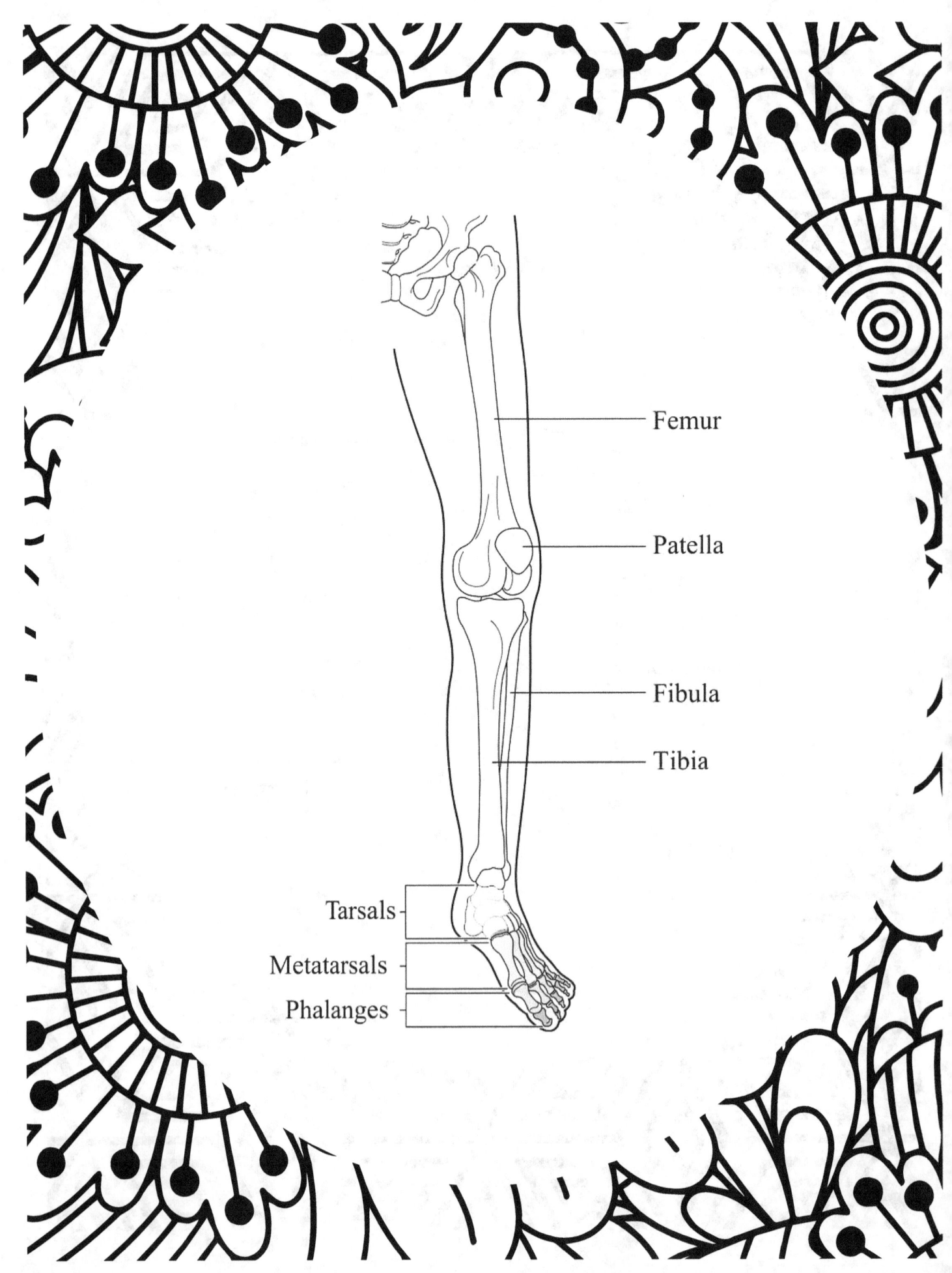

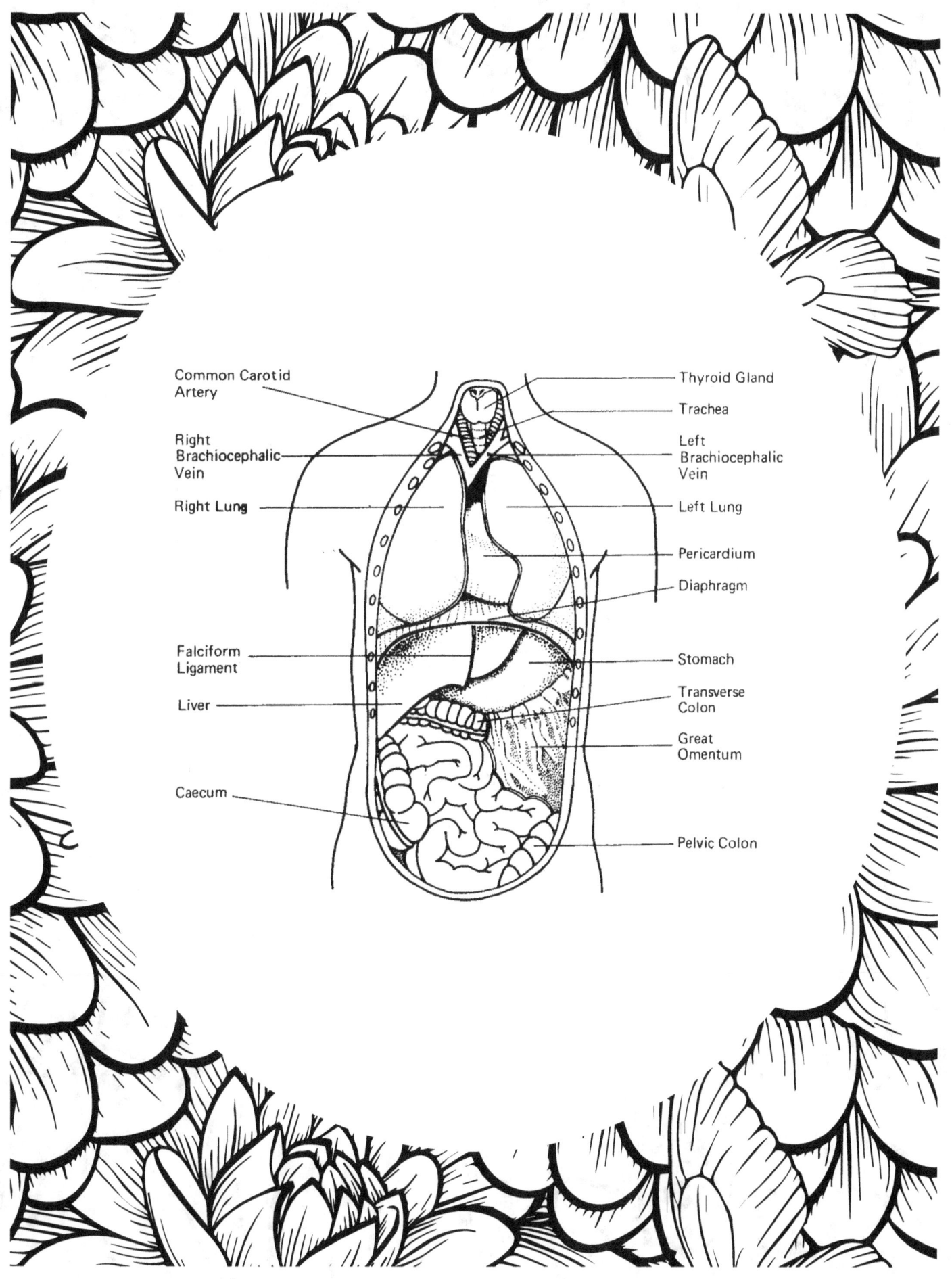

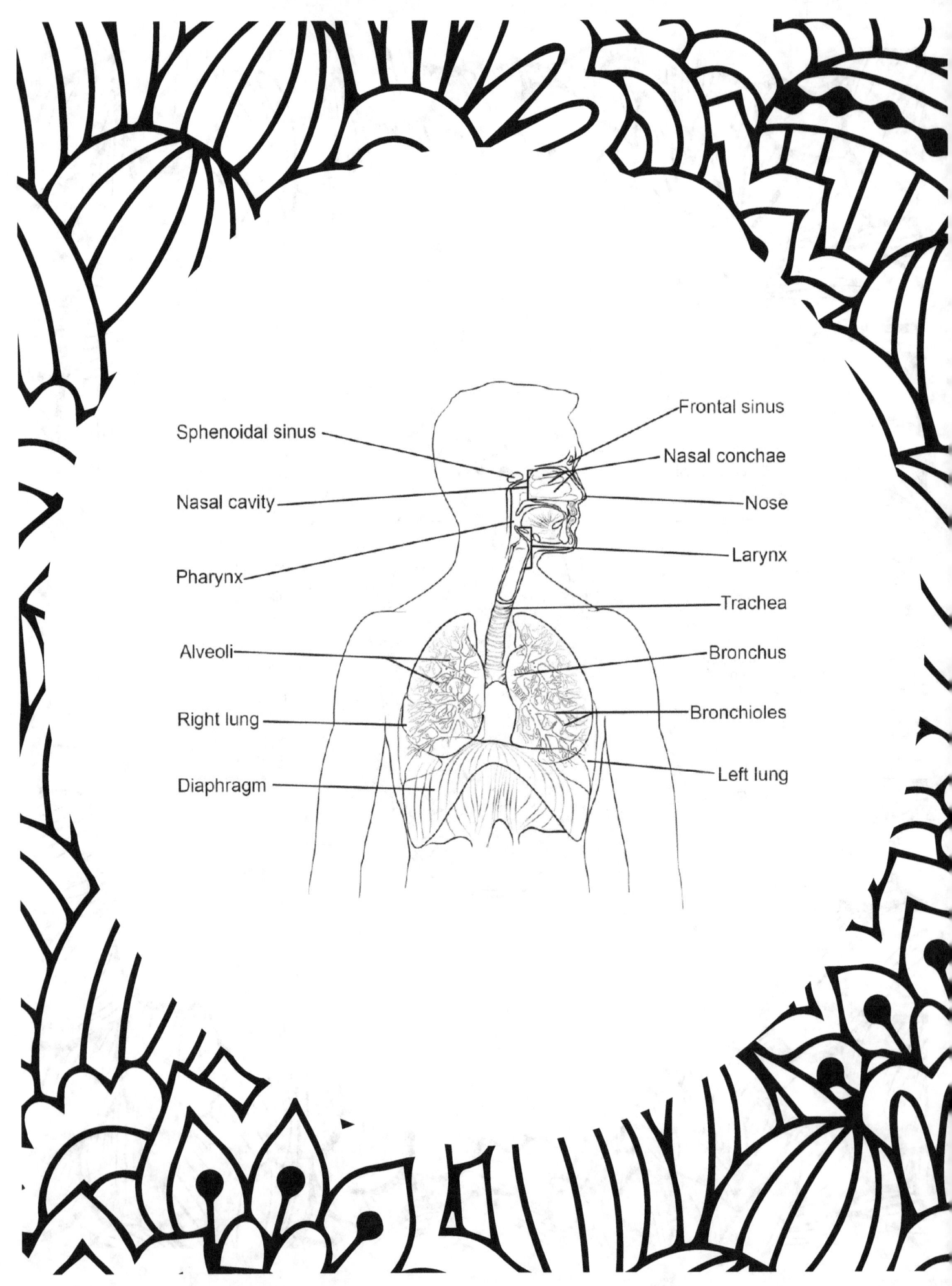

Color the Structures Connected to Liver Function

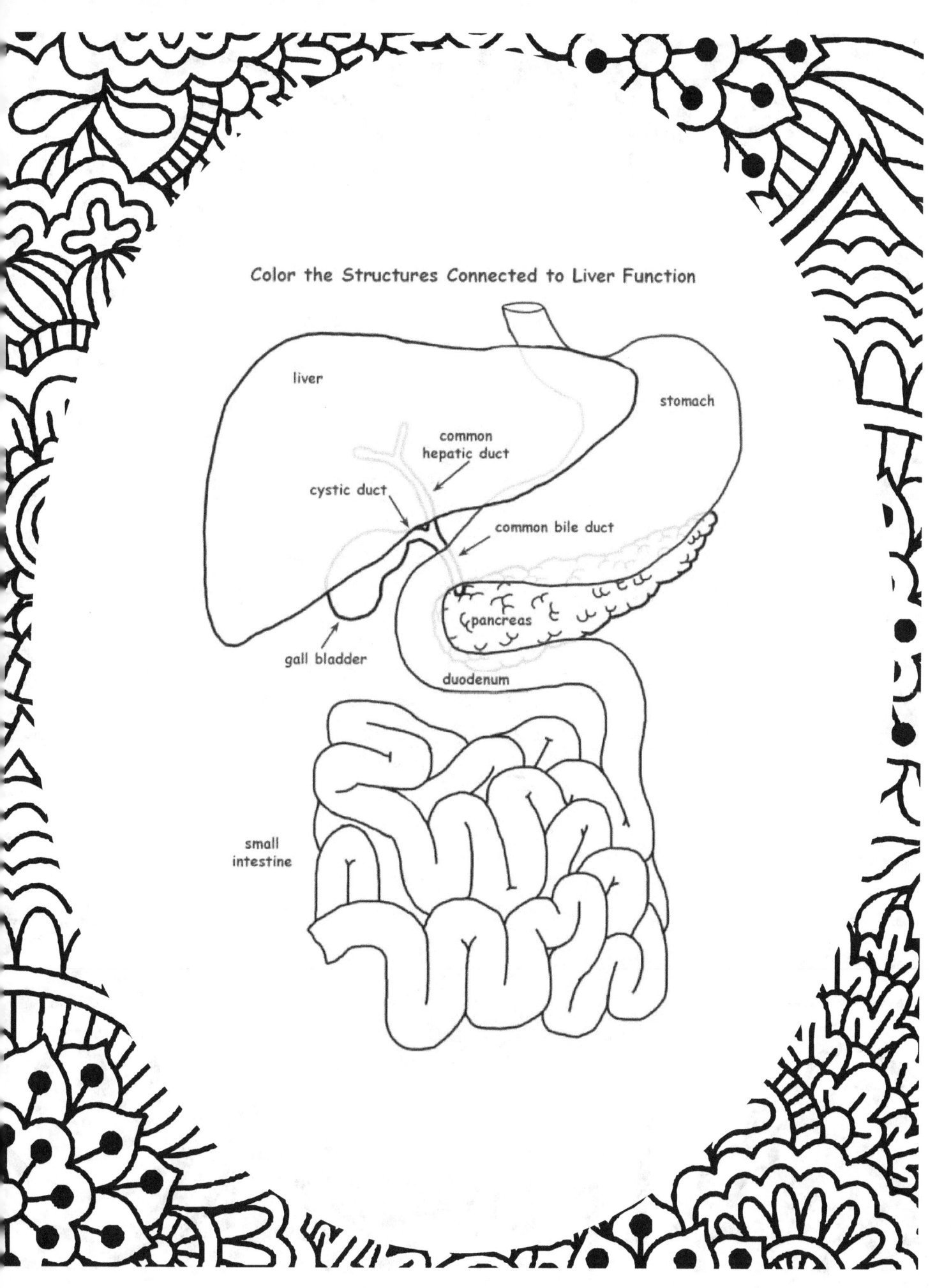

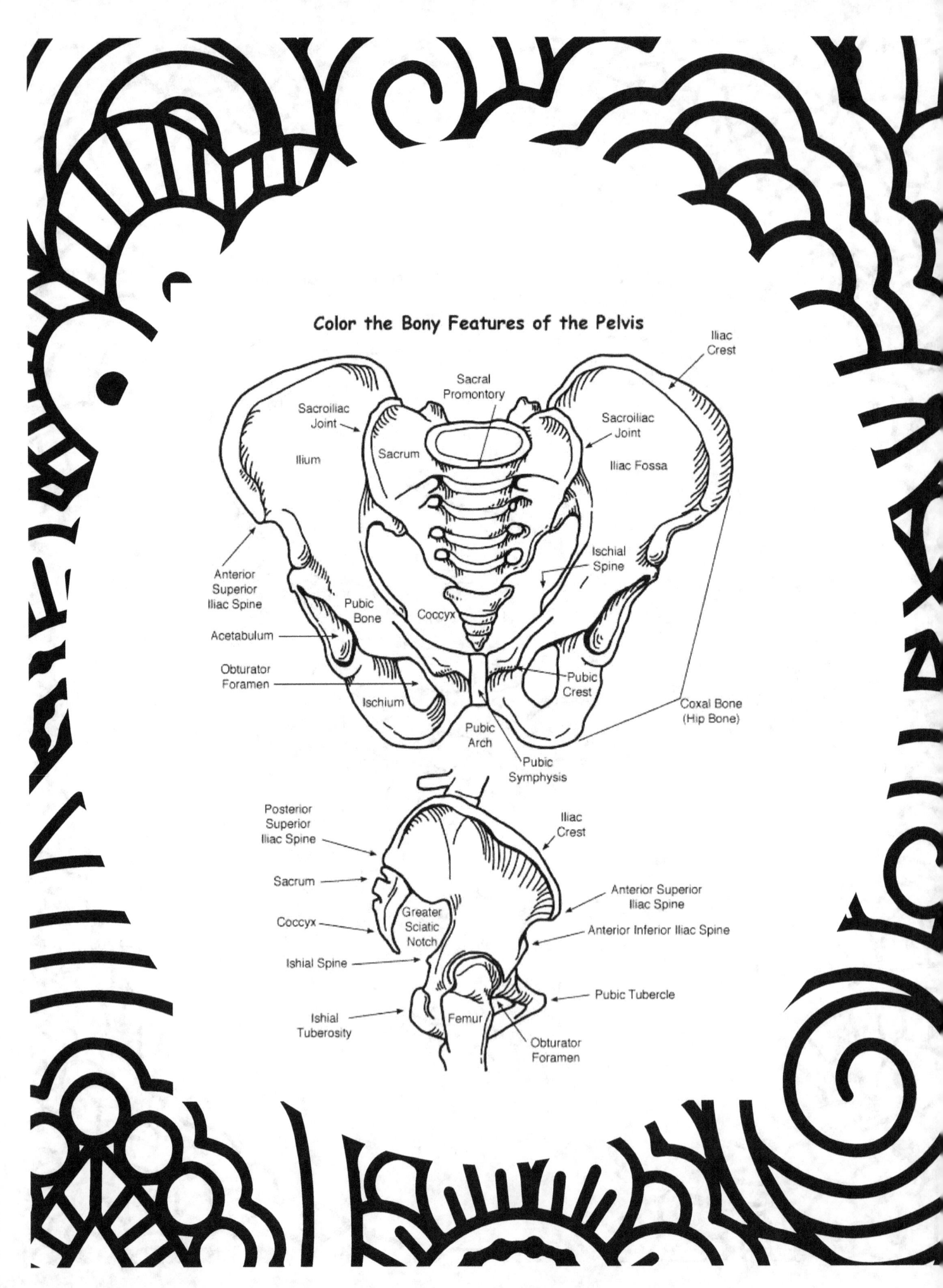

Color the Bony Features of the Pelvis

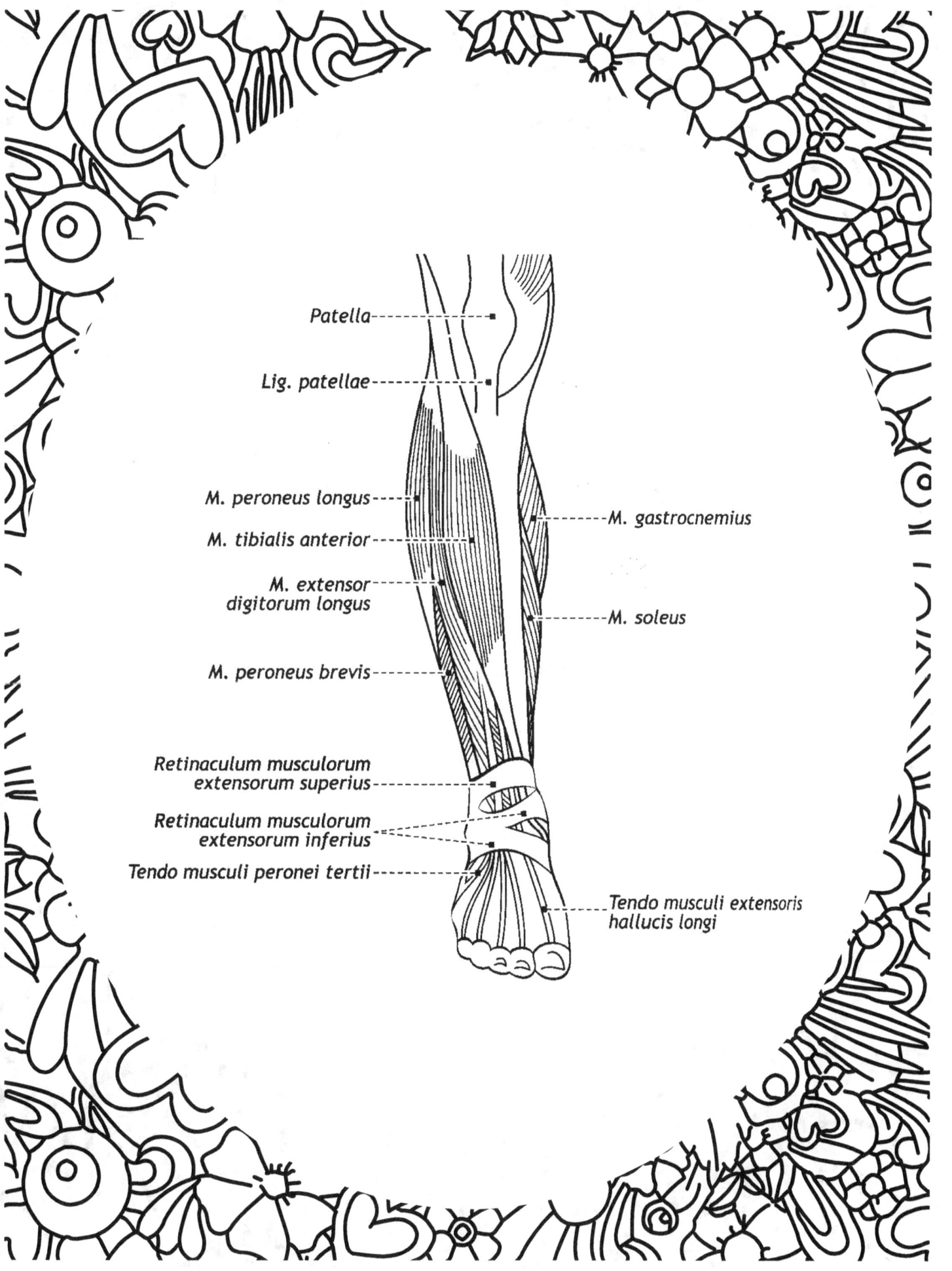

Patella

Lig. patellae

M. peroneus longus

M. tibialis anterior

M. extensor
digitorum longus

M. peroneus brevis

Retinaculum musculorum
extensorum superius

Retinaculum musculorum
extensorum inferius

Tendo musculi peronei tertii

M. gastrocnemius

M. soleus

Tendo musculi extensoris
hallucis longi

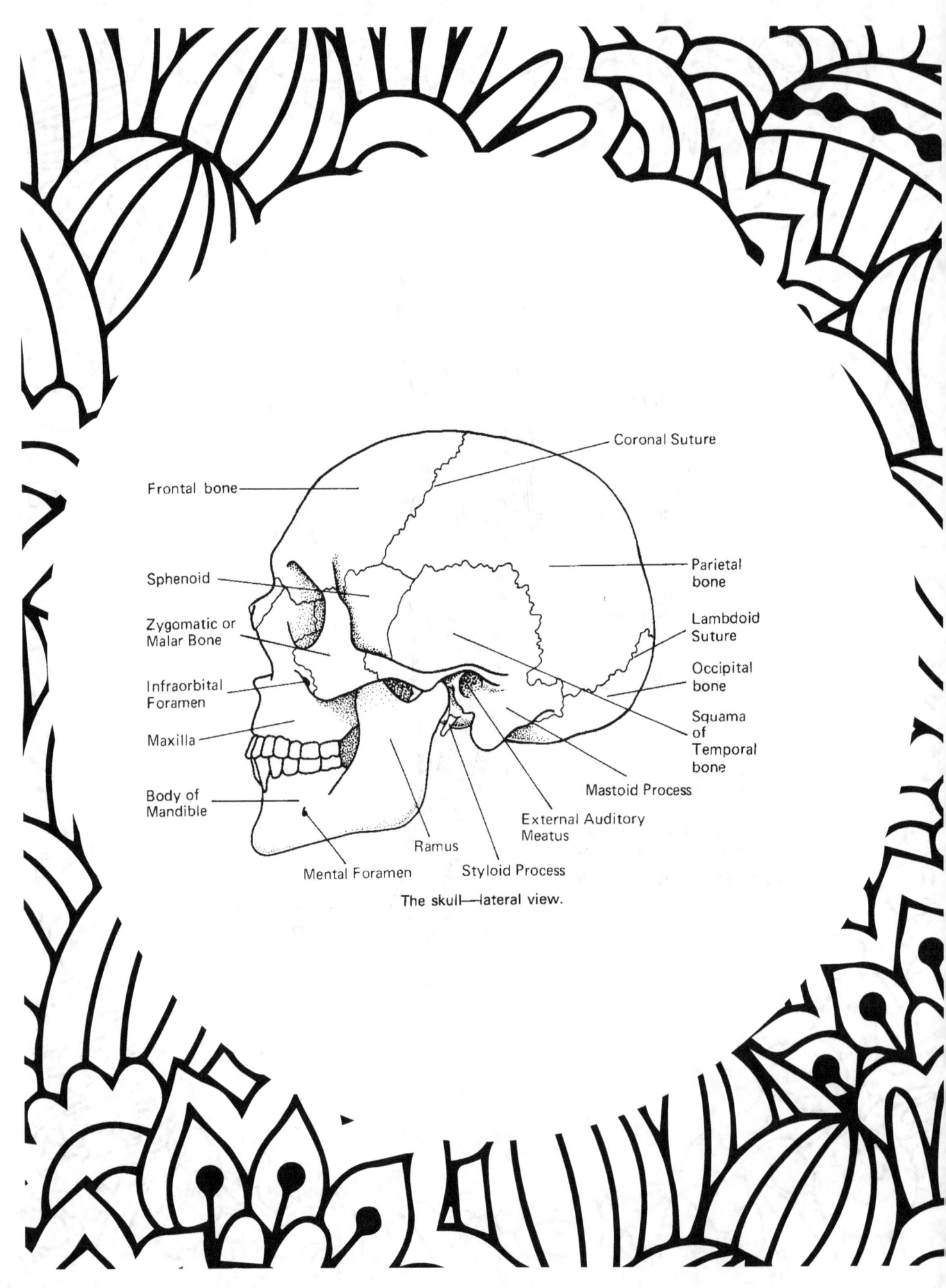

The skull—lateral view.

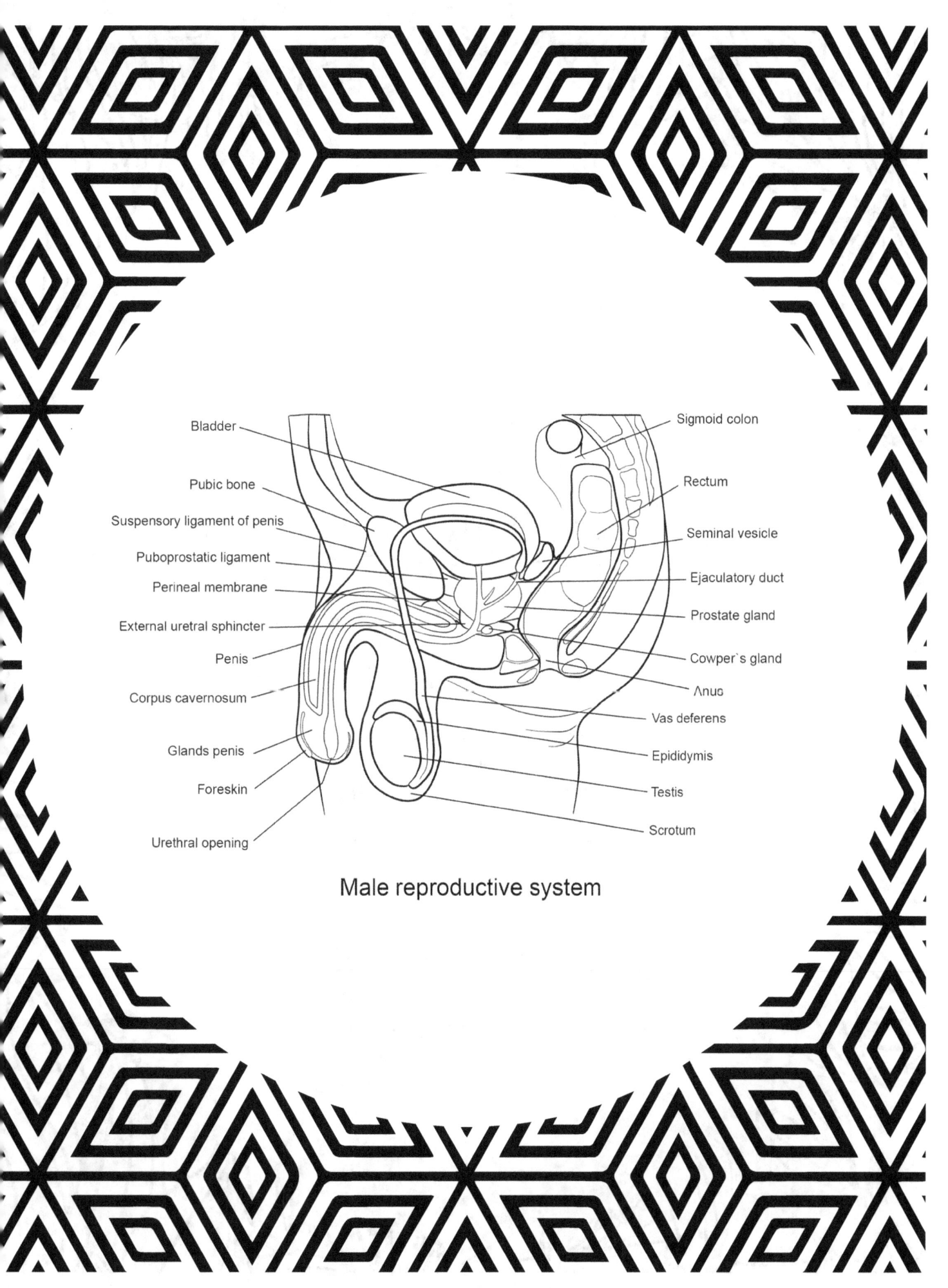

Male reproductive system

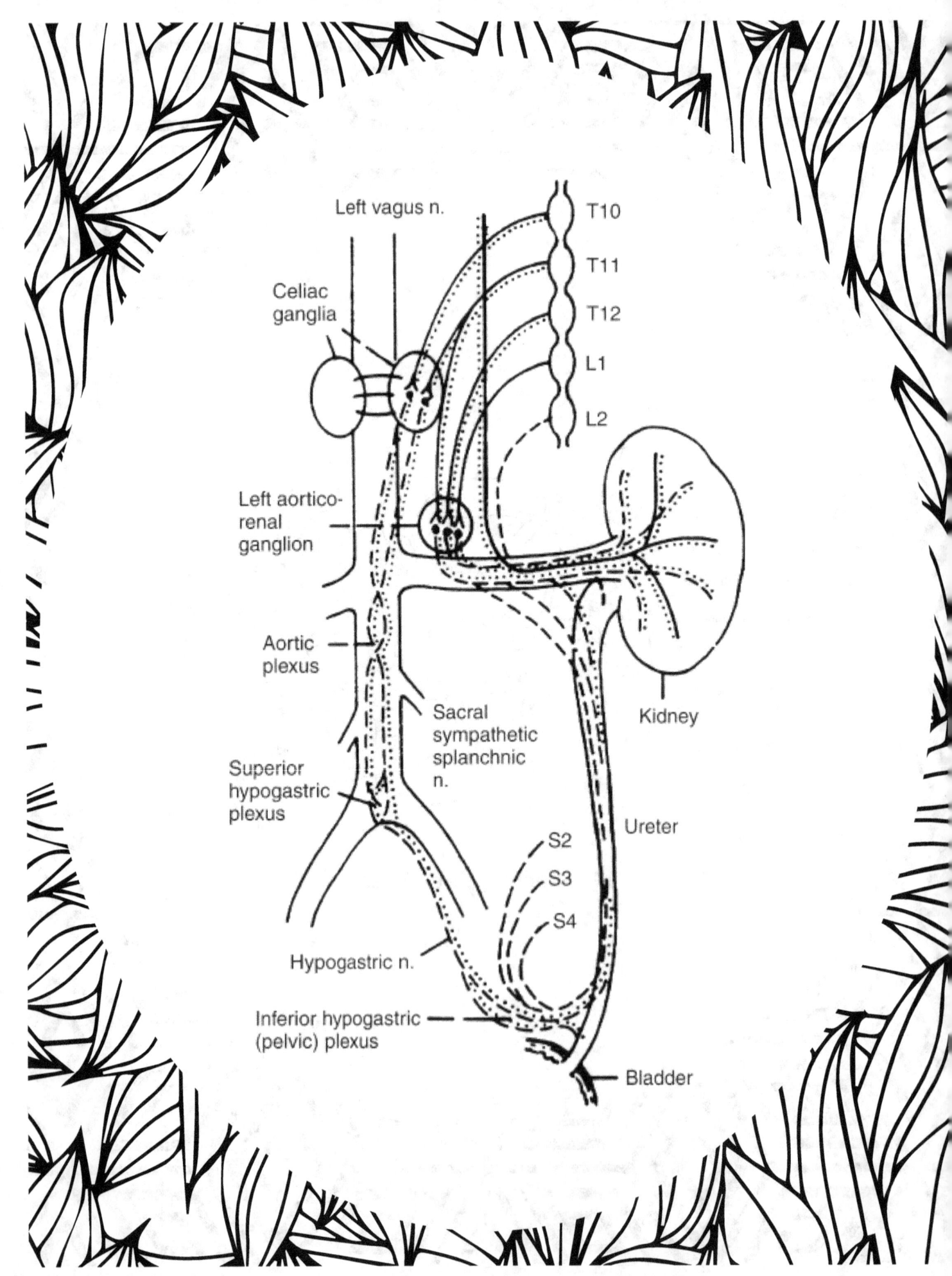

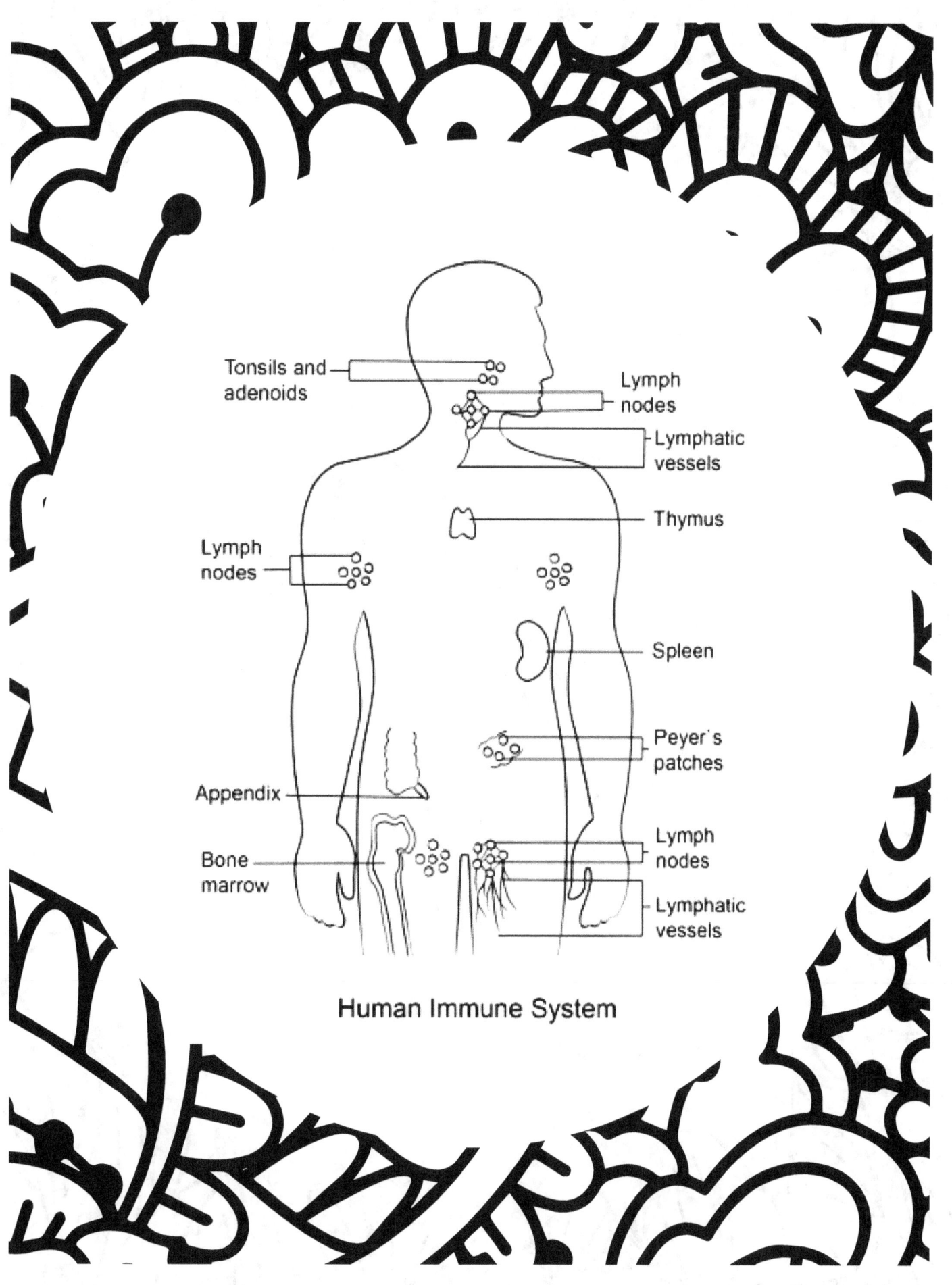

Human Immune System

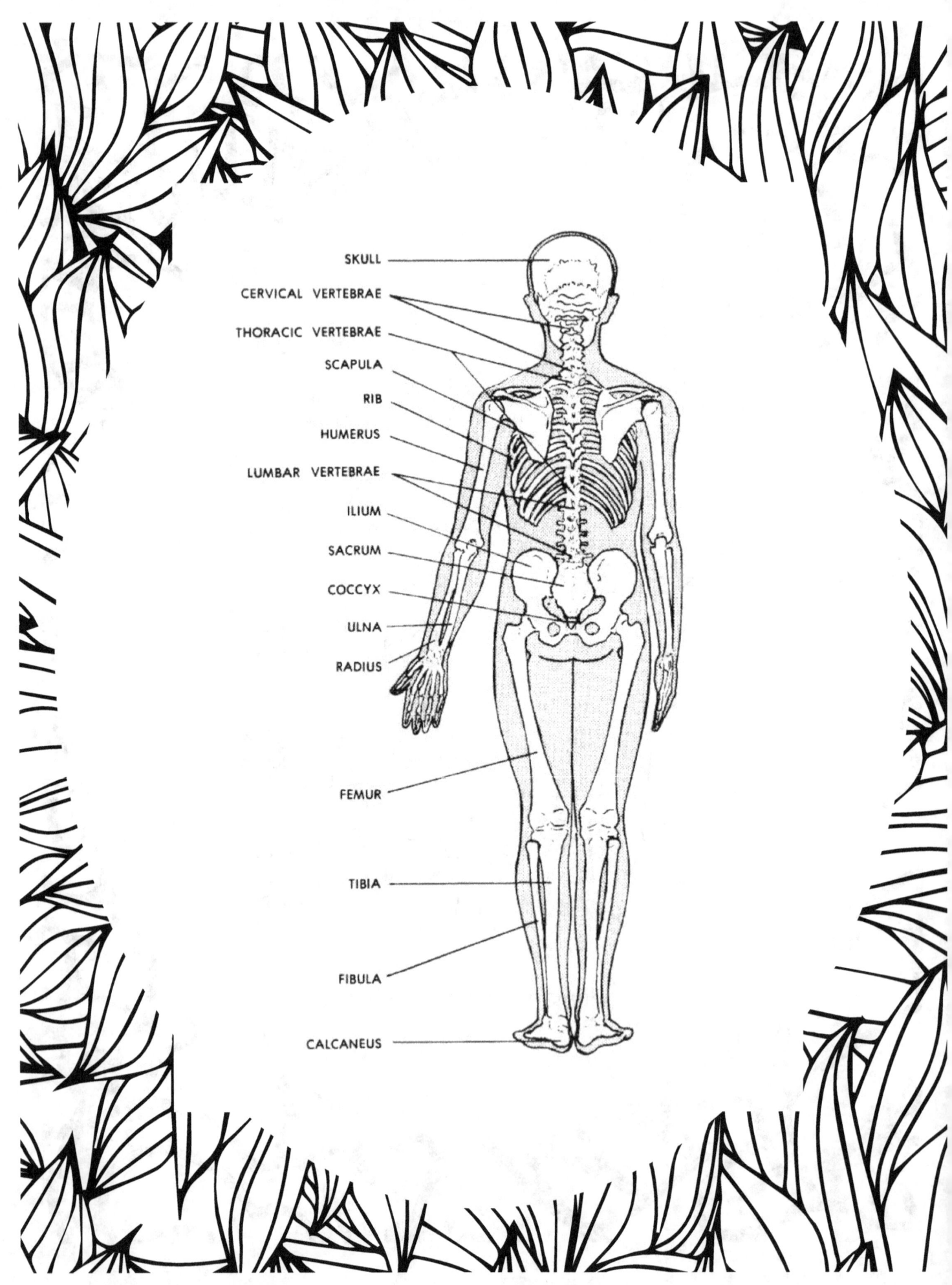

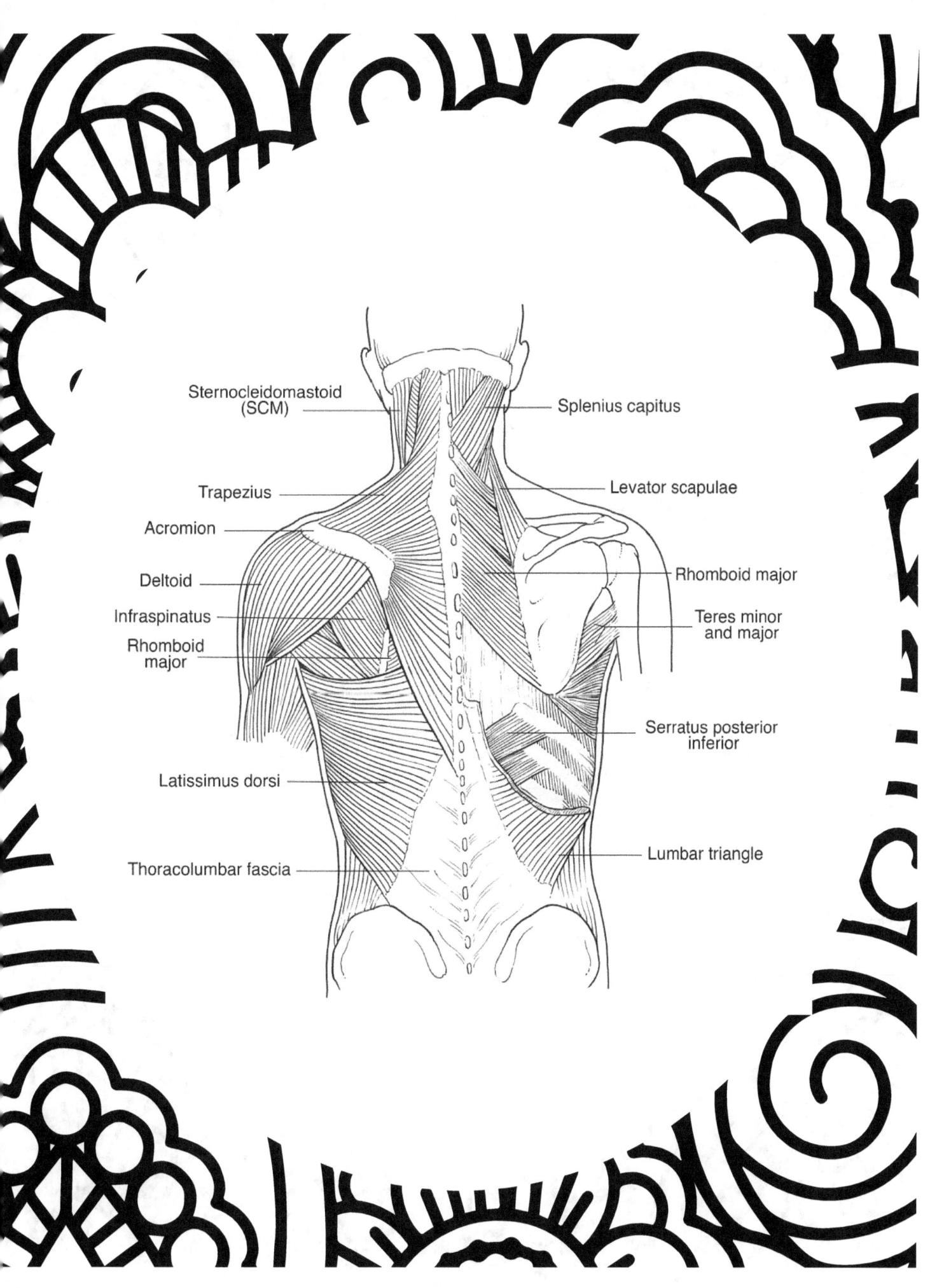

Coronary Arteries

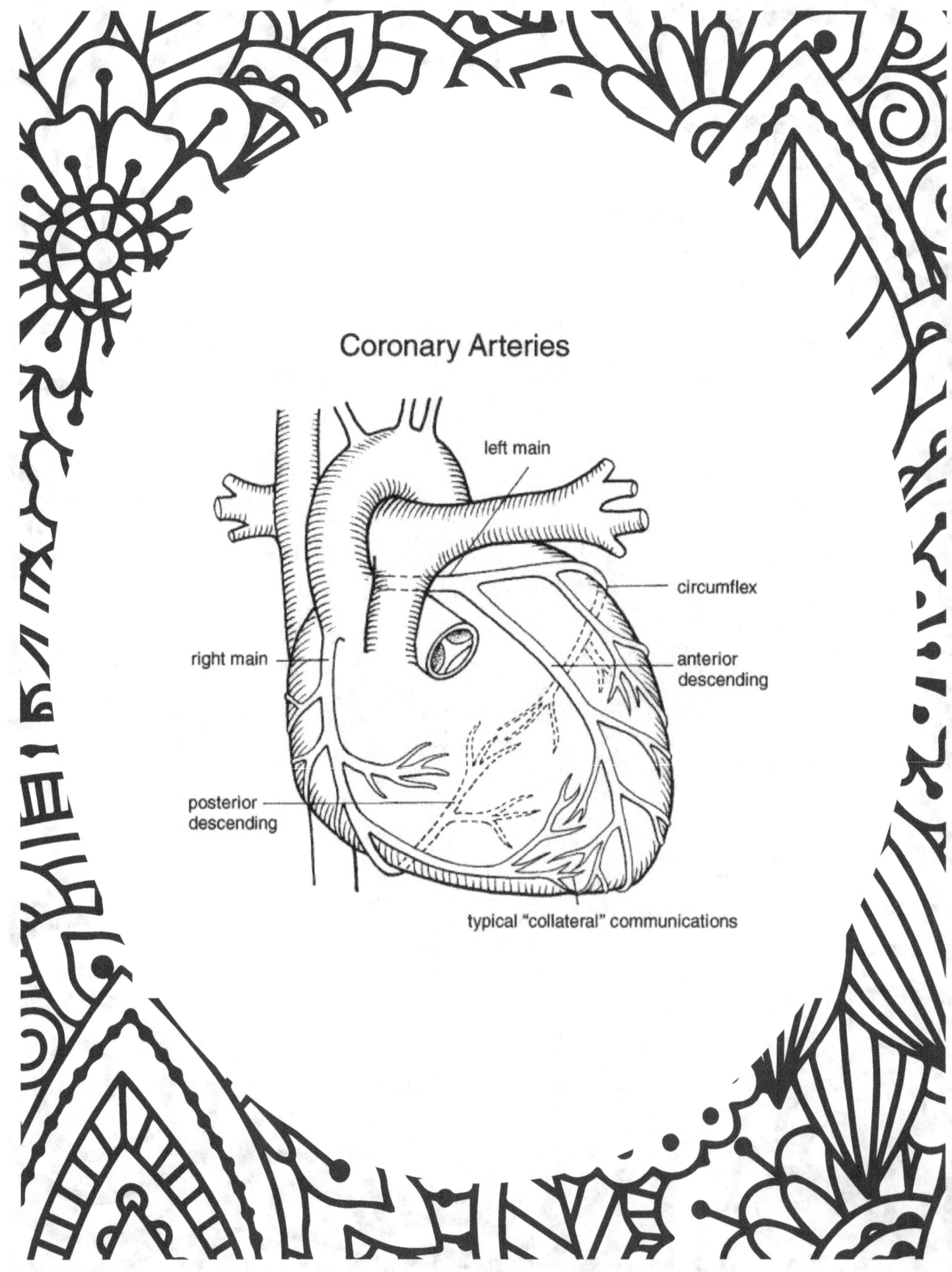

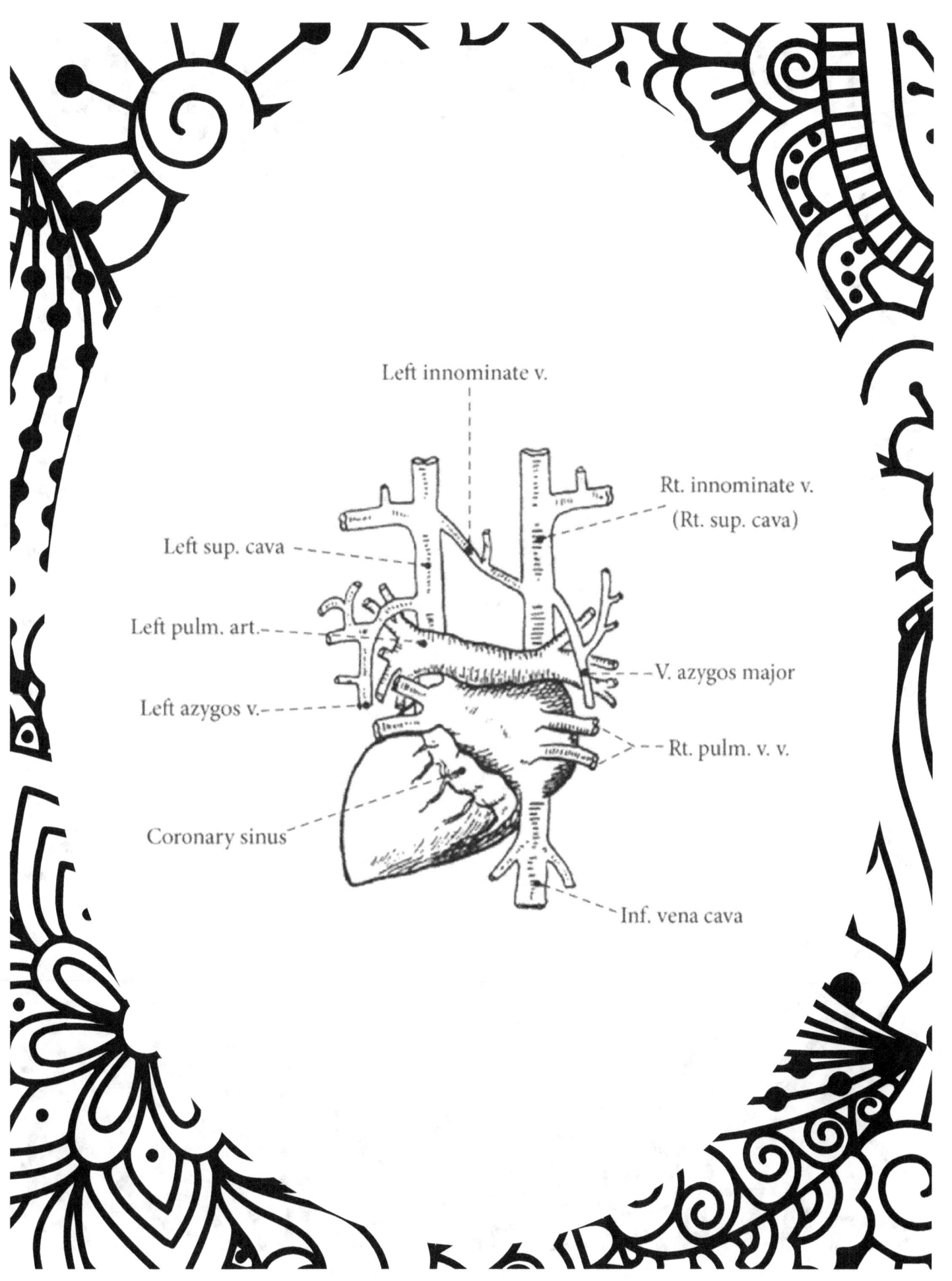

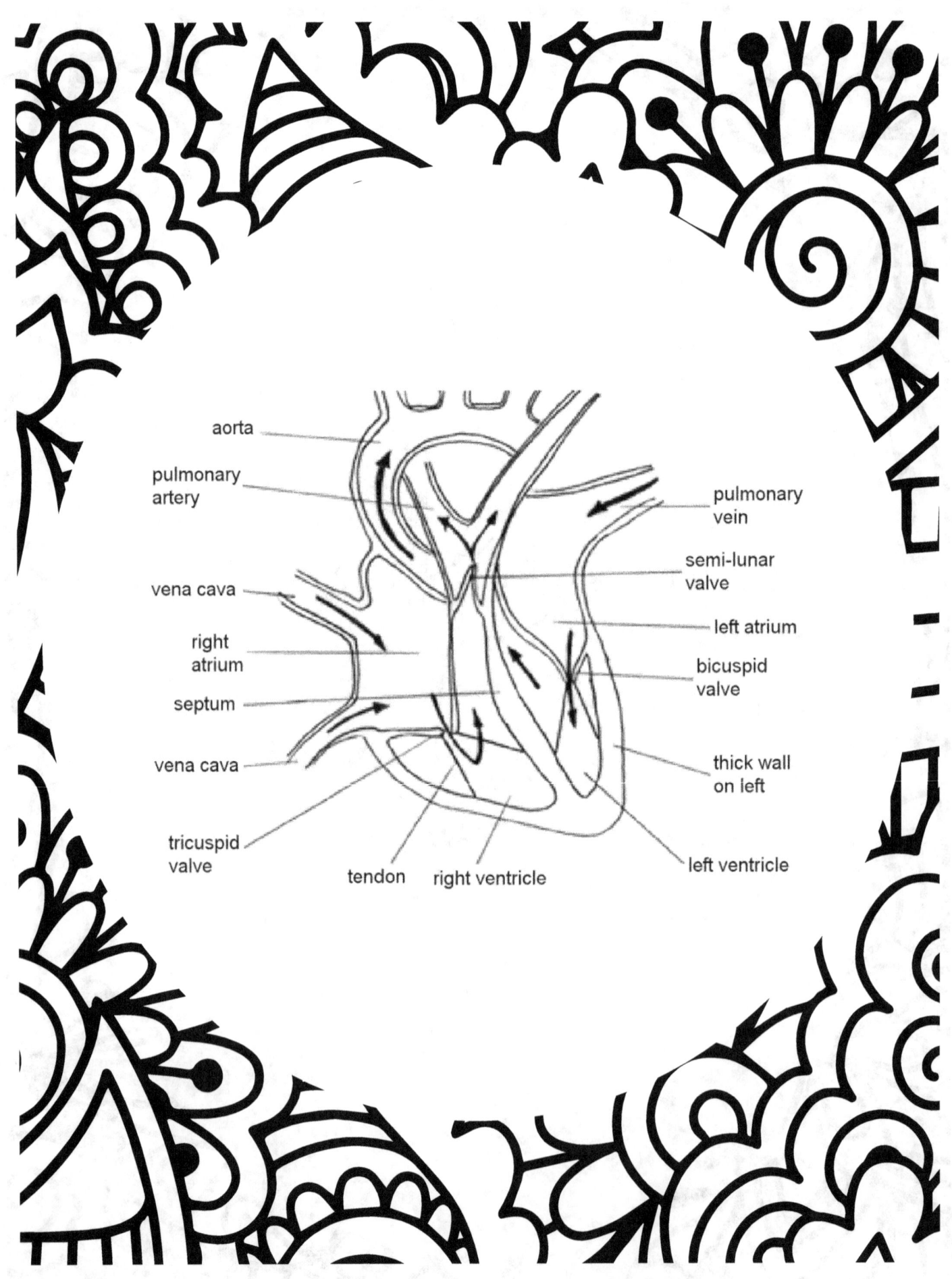

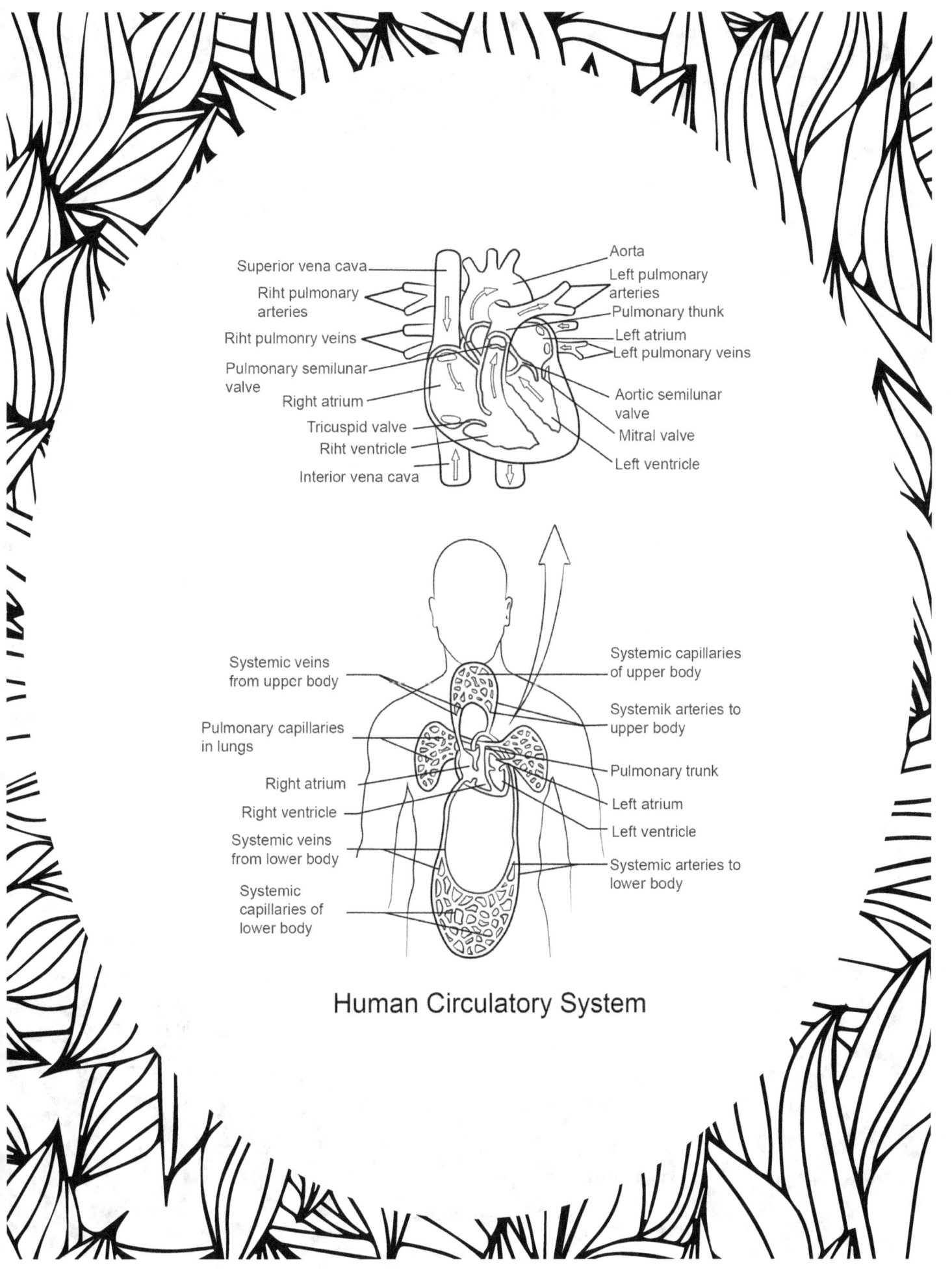

Human Circulatory System

parts of an ear

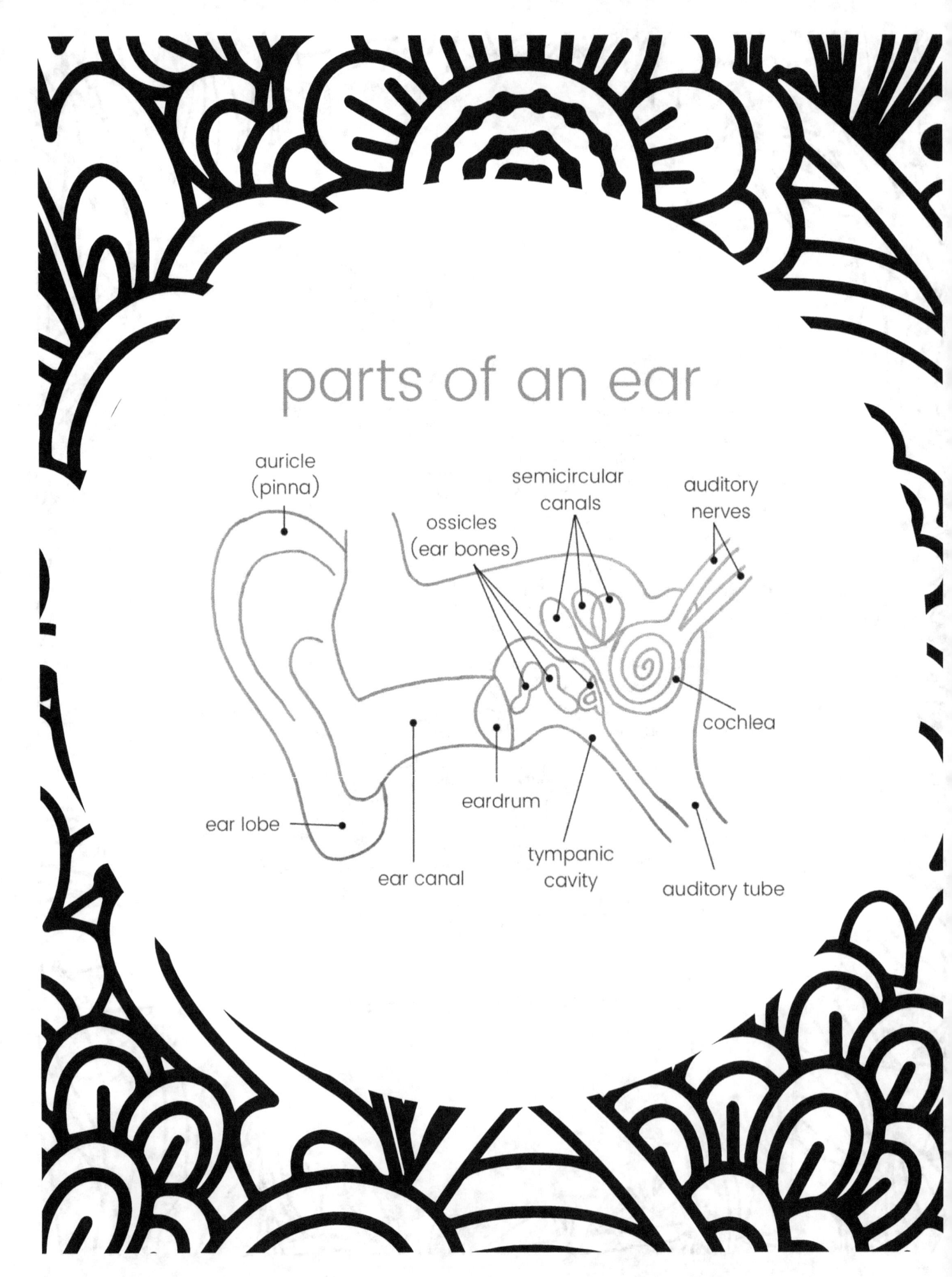

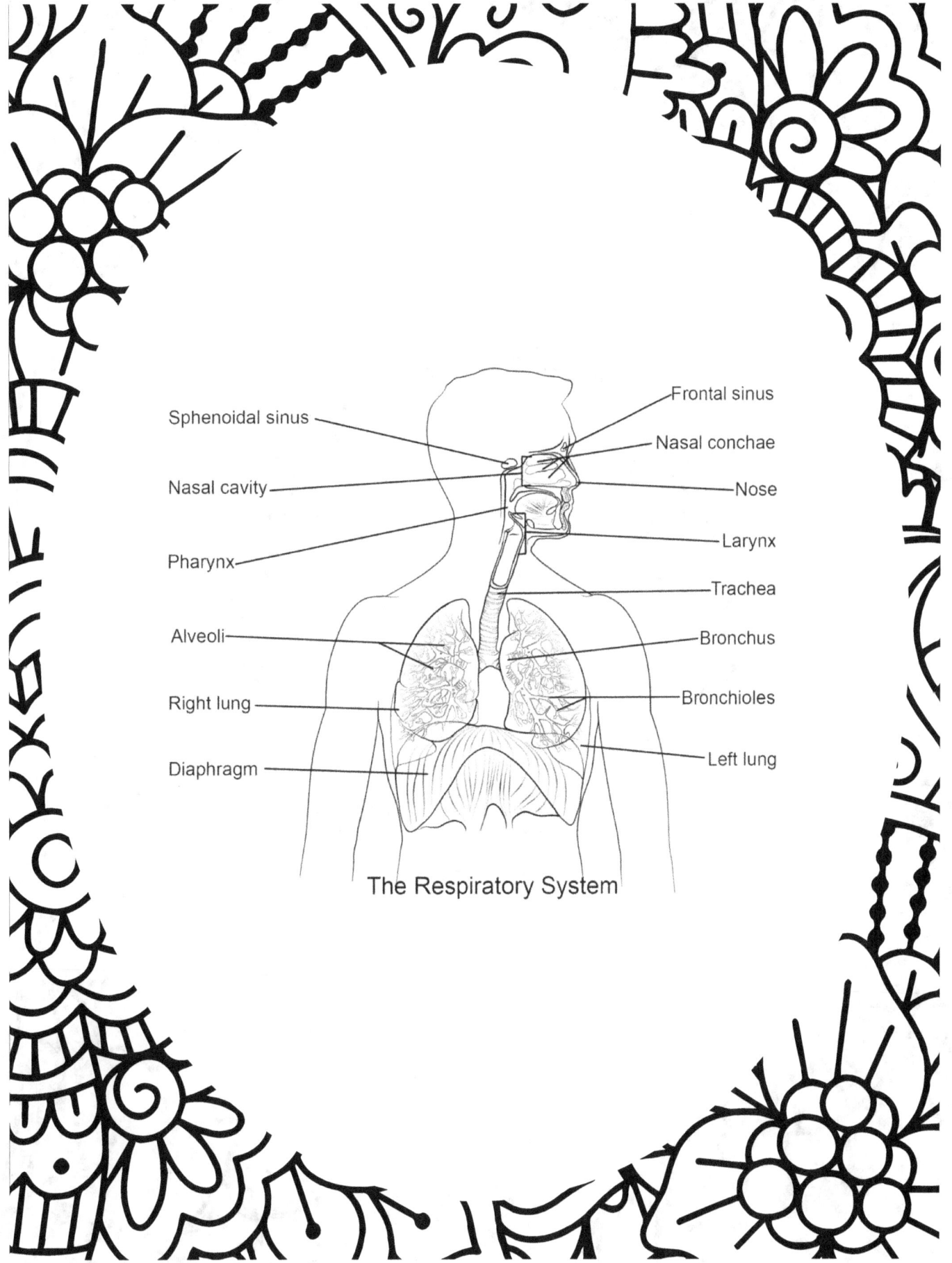

The Respiratory System

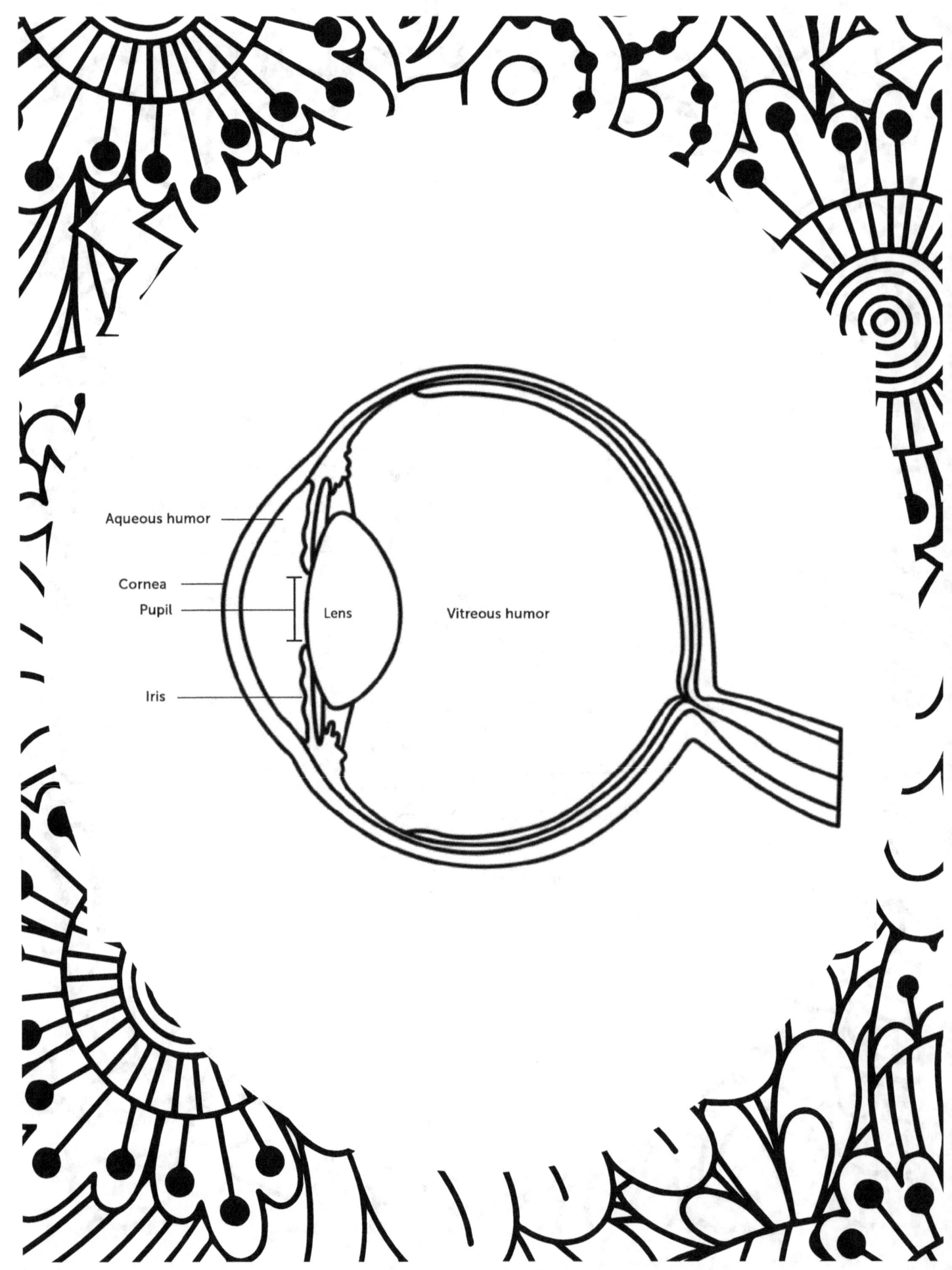

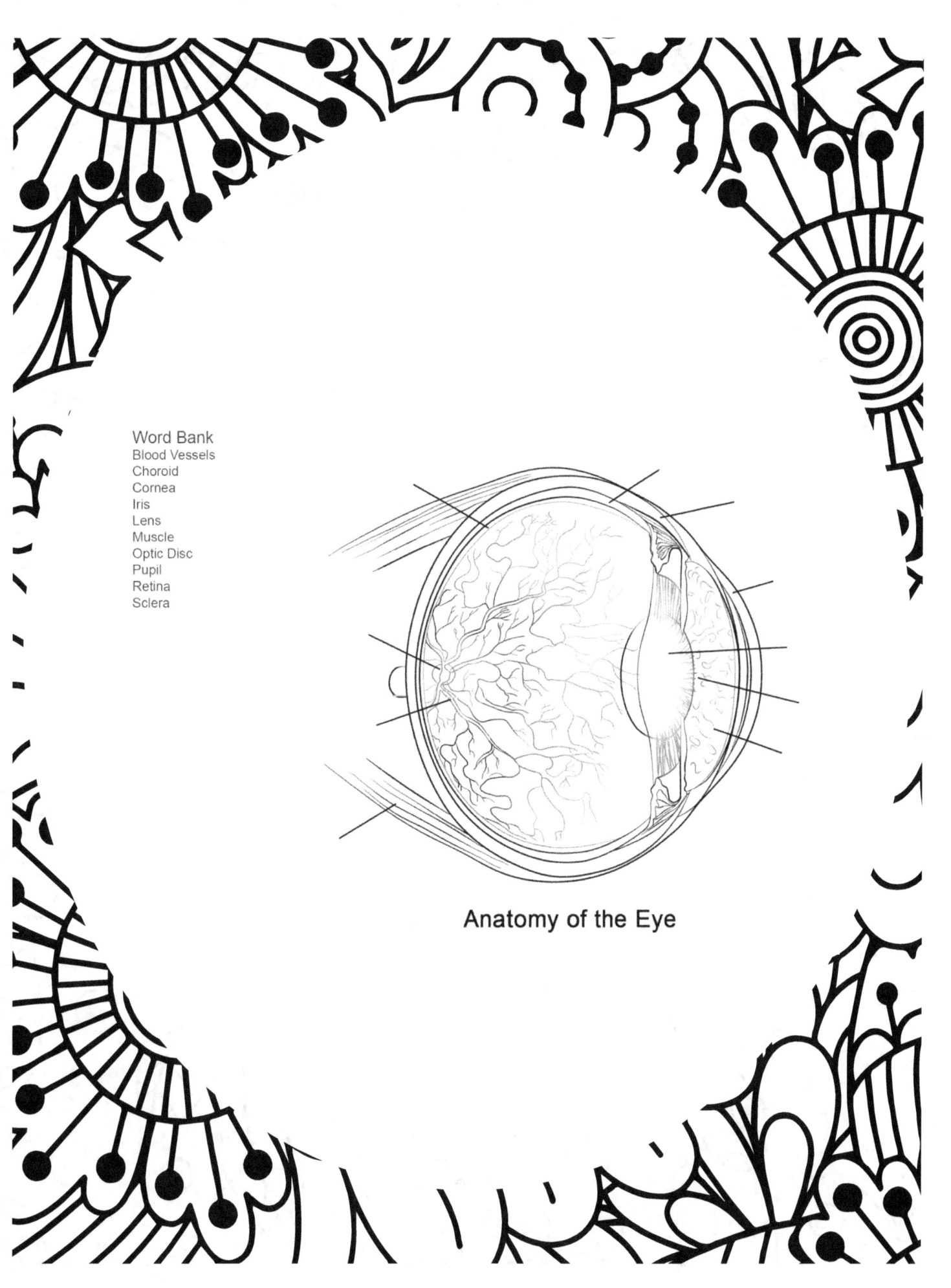

Word Bank
Blood Vessels
Choroid
Cornea
Iris
Lens
Muscle
Optic Disc
Pupil
Retina
Sclera

Anatomy of the Eye

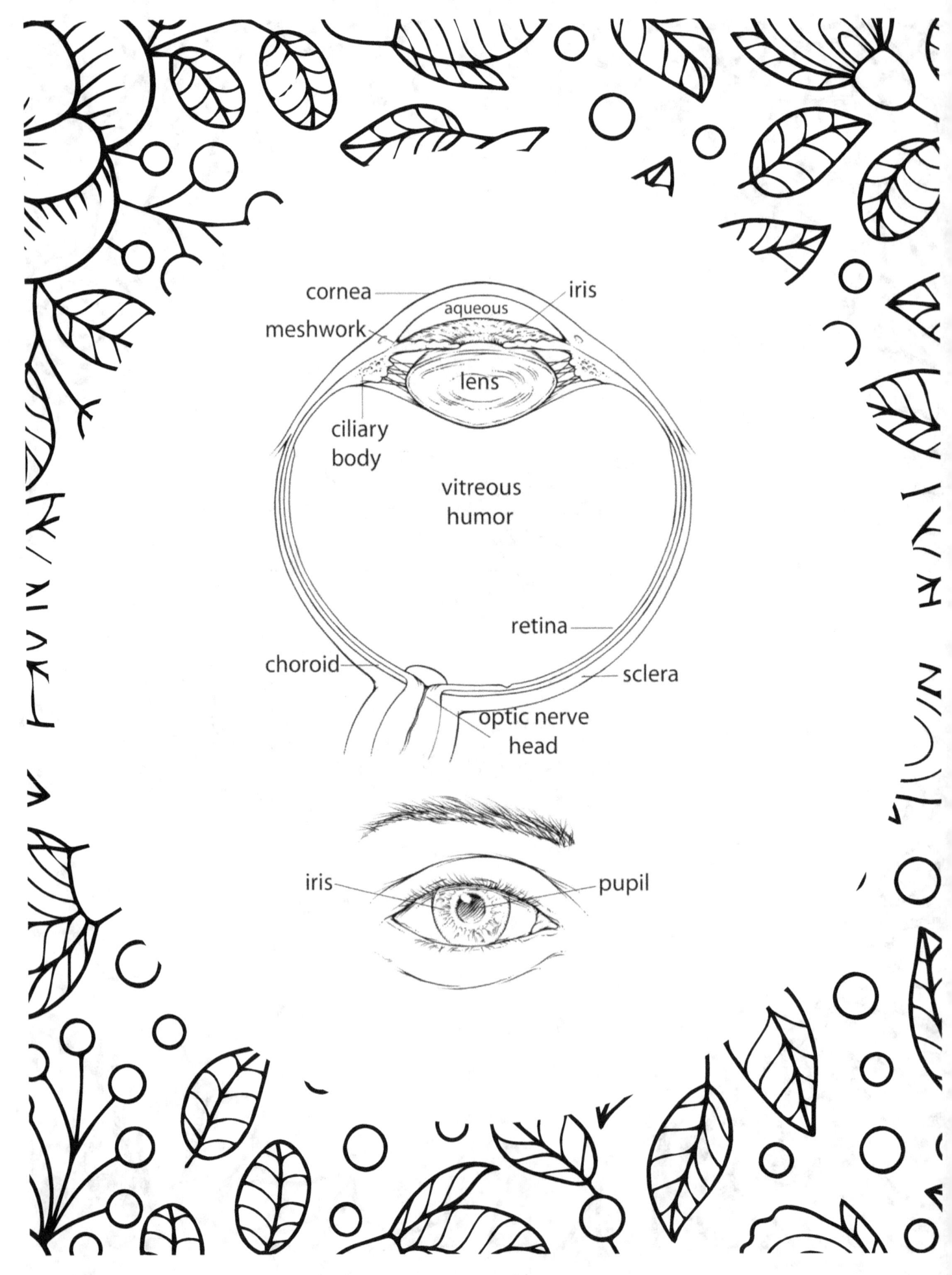

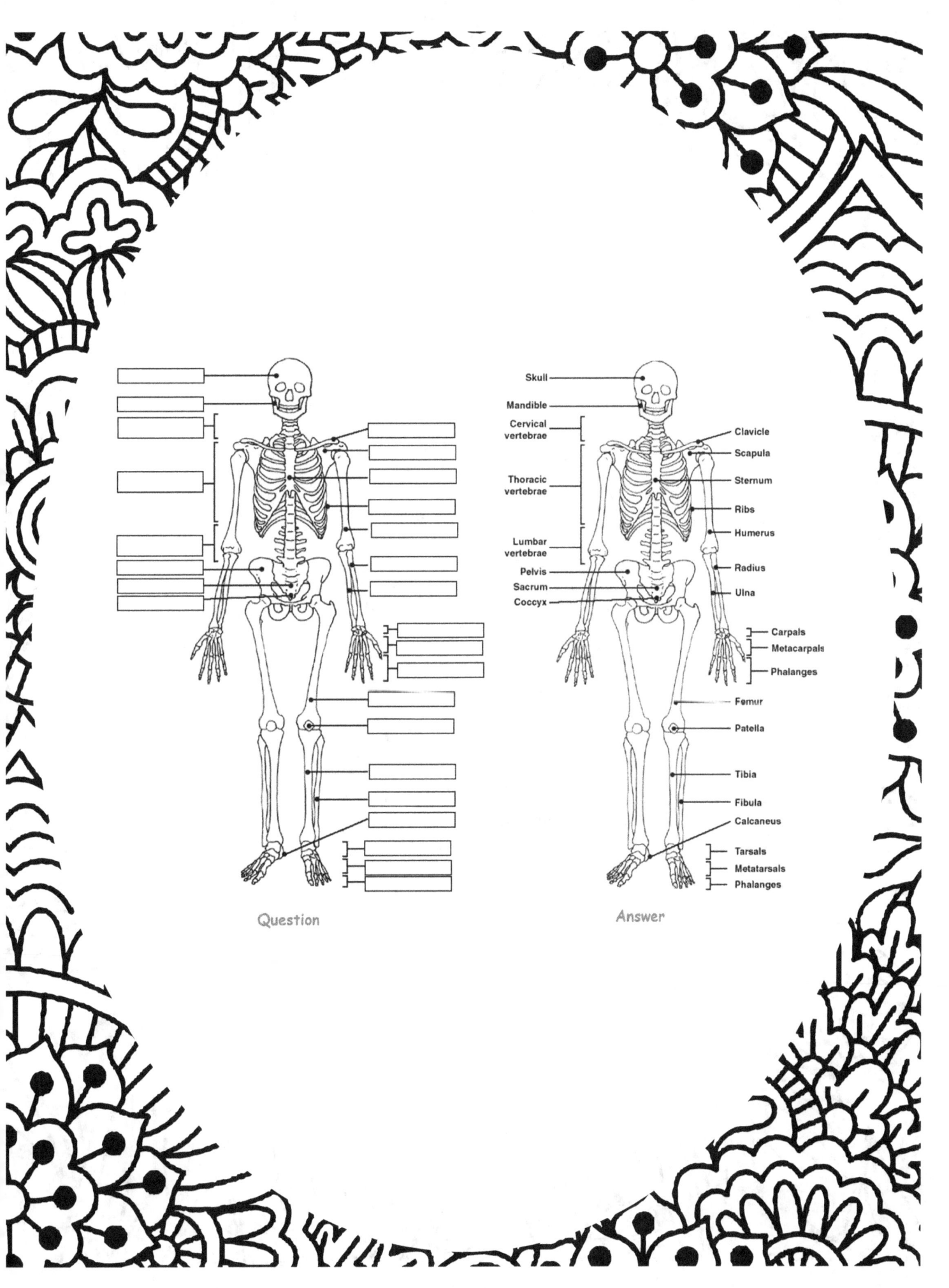

Question

Answer

Skull
Mandible
Cervical vertebrae
Thoracic vertebrae
Lumbar vertebrae
Pelvis
Sacrum
Coccyx
Clavicle
Scapula
Sternum
Ribs
Humerus
Radius
Ulna
Carpals
Metacarpals
Phalanges
Femur
Patella
Tibia
Fibula
Calcaneus
Tarsals
Metatarsals
Phalanges

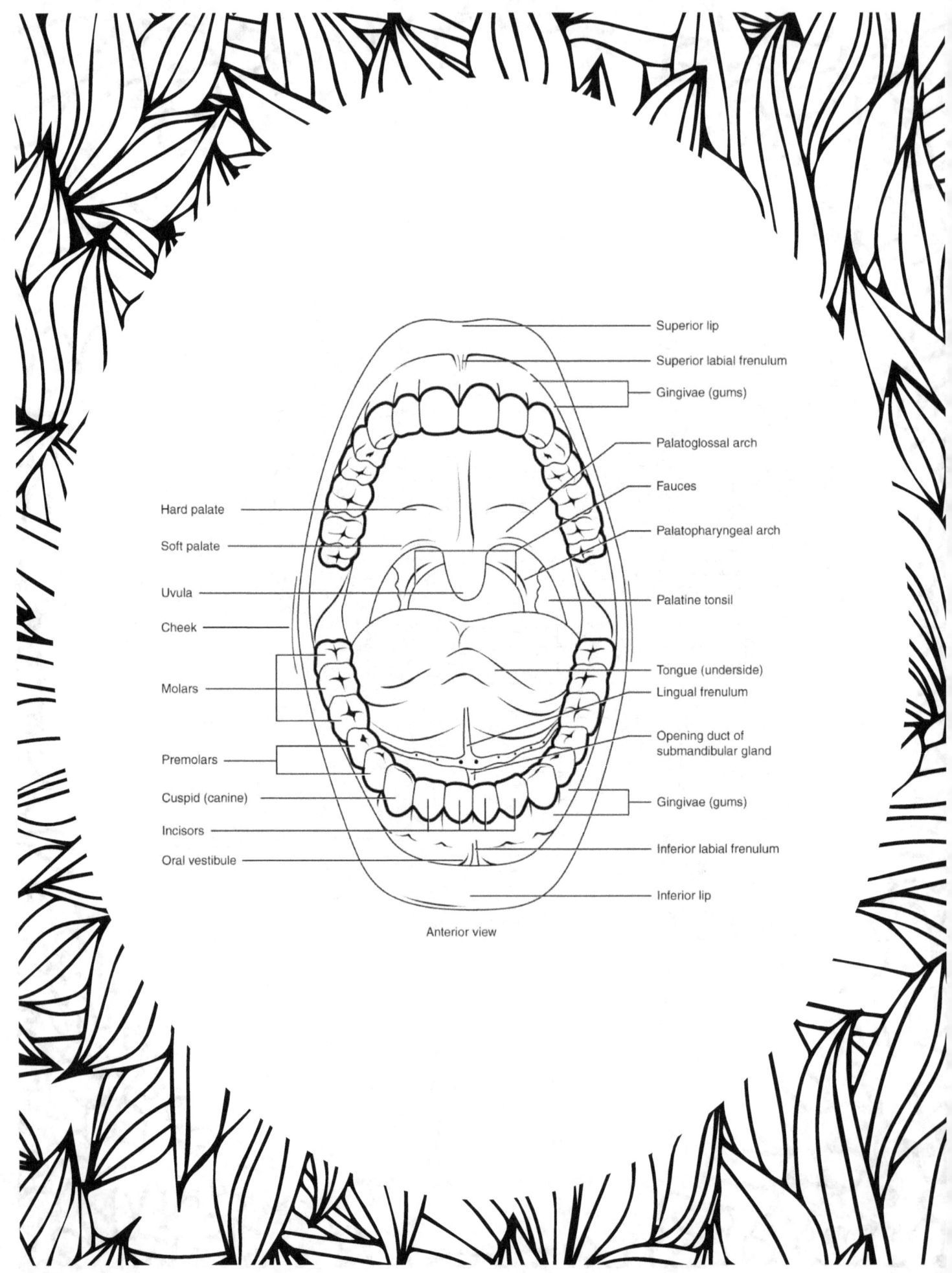

Superior lip

Superior labial frenulum

Gingivae (gums)

Palatoglossal arch

Fauces

Palatopharyngeal arch

Palatine tonsil

Tongue (underside)

Lingual frenulum

Opening duct of
submandibular gland

Gingivae (gums)

Inferior labial frenulum

Inferior lip

Hard palate

Soft palate

Uvula

Cheek

Molars

Premolars

Cuspid (canine)

Incisors

Oral vestibule

Anterior view

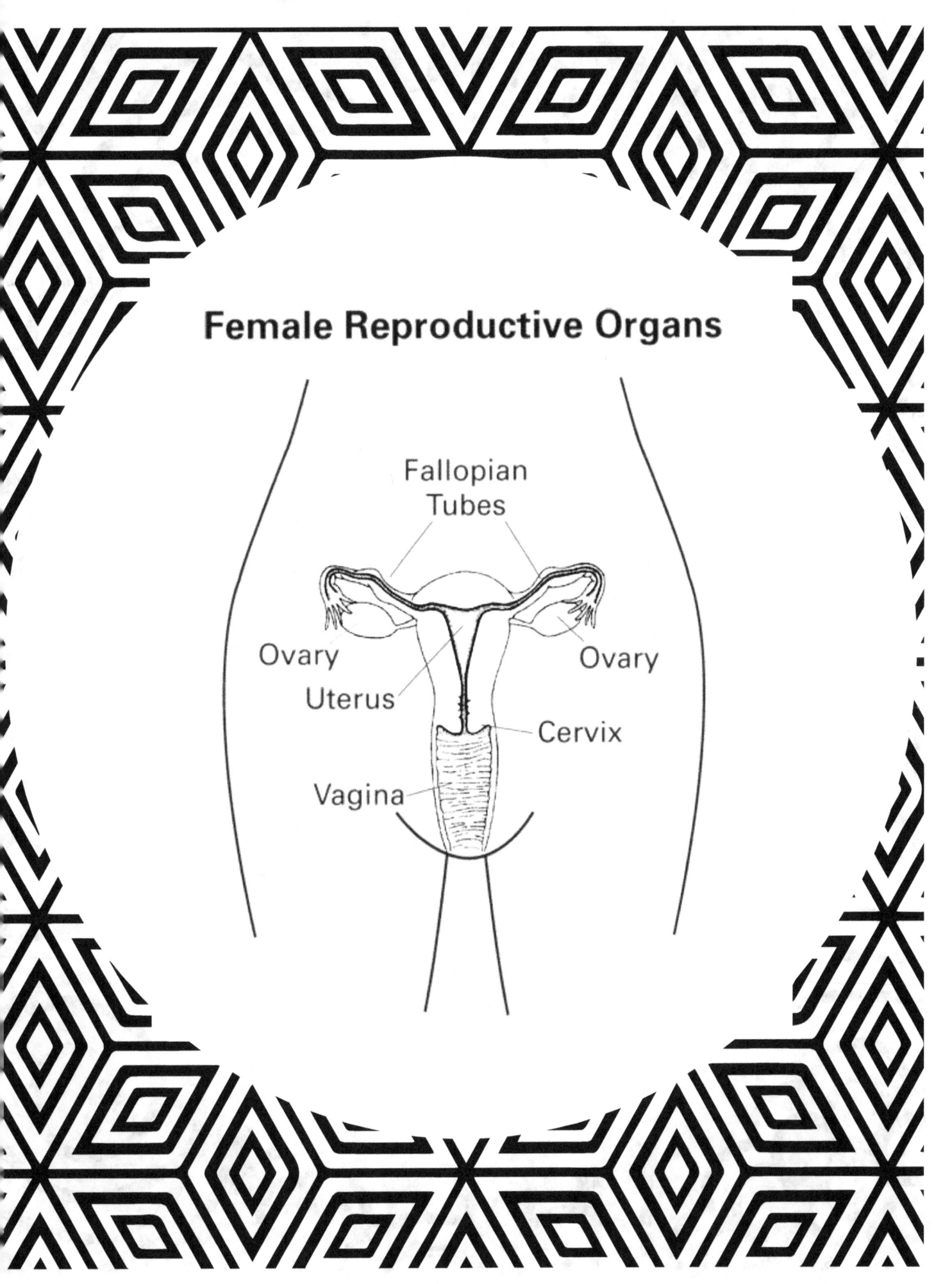

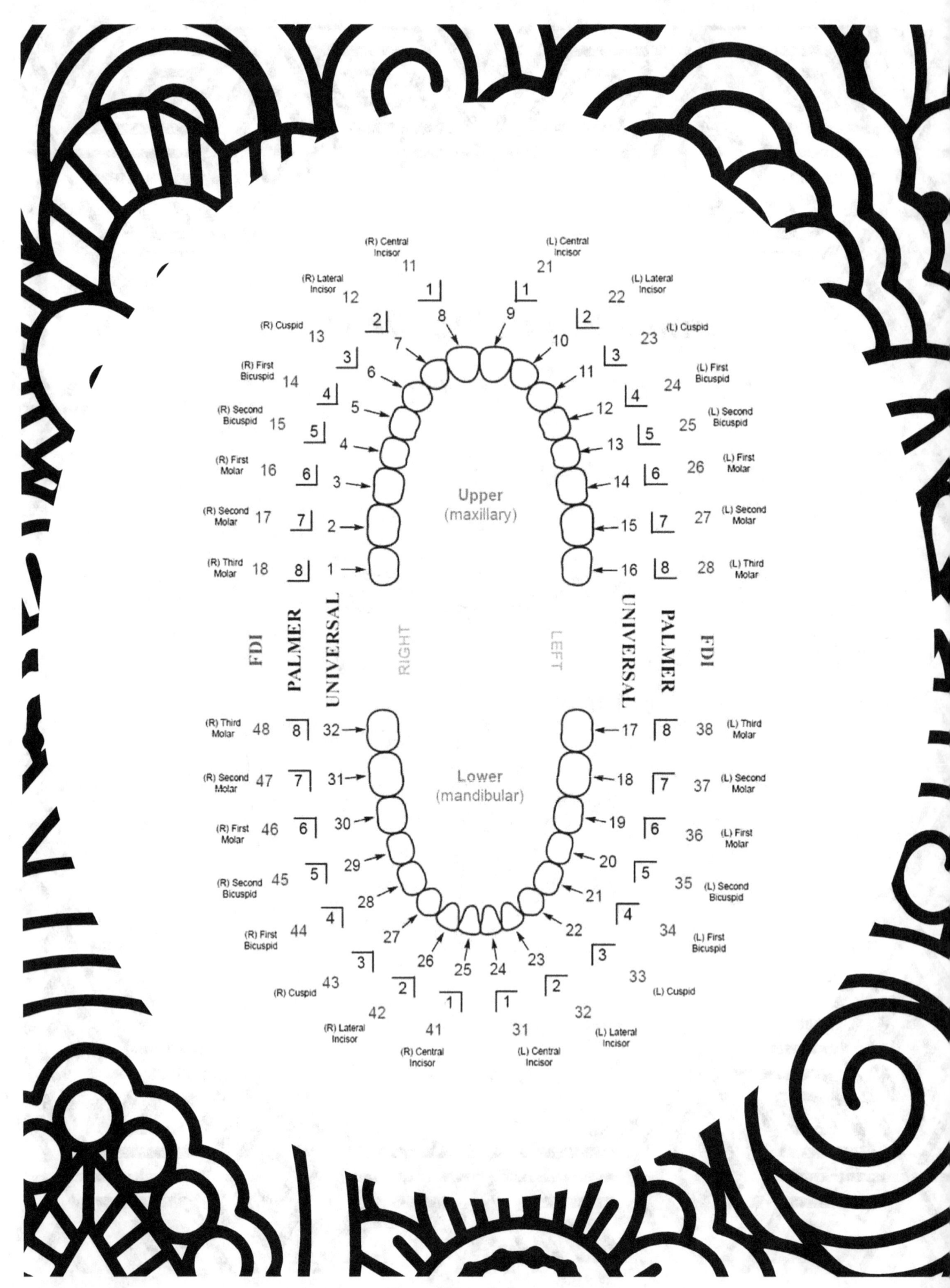

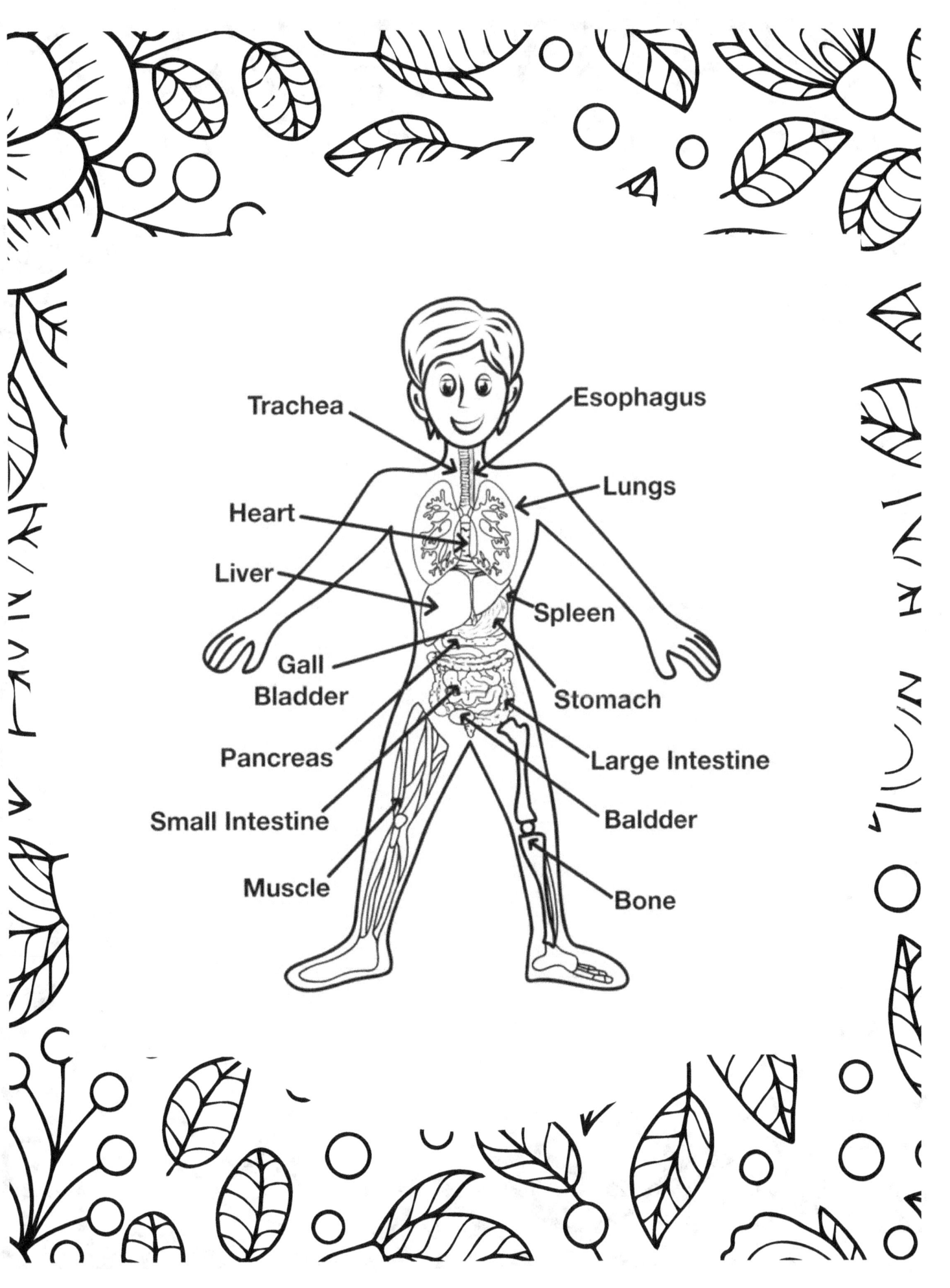

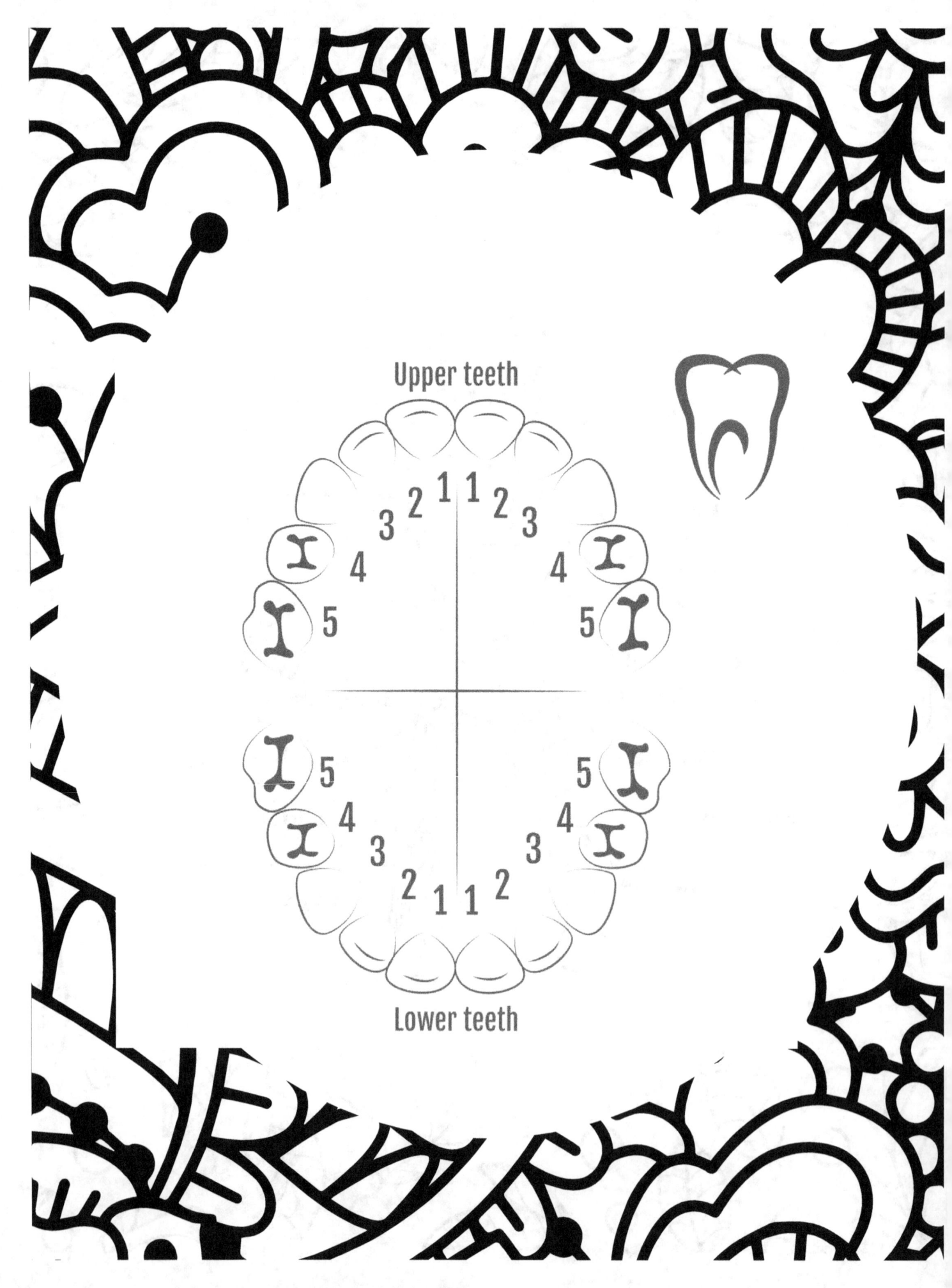

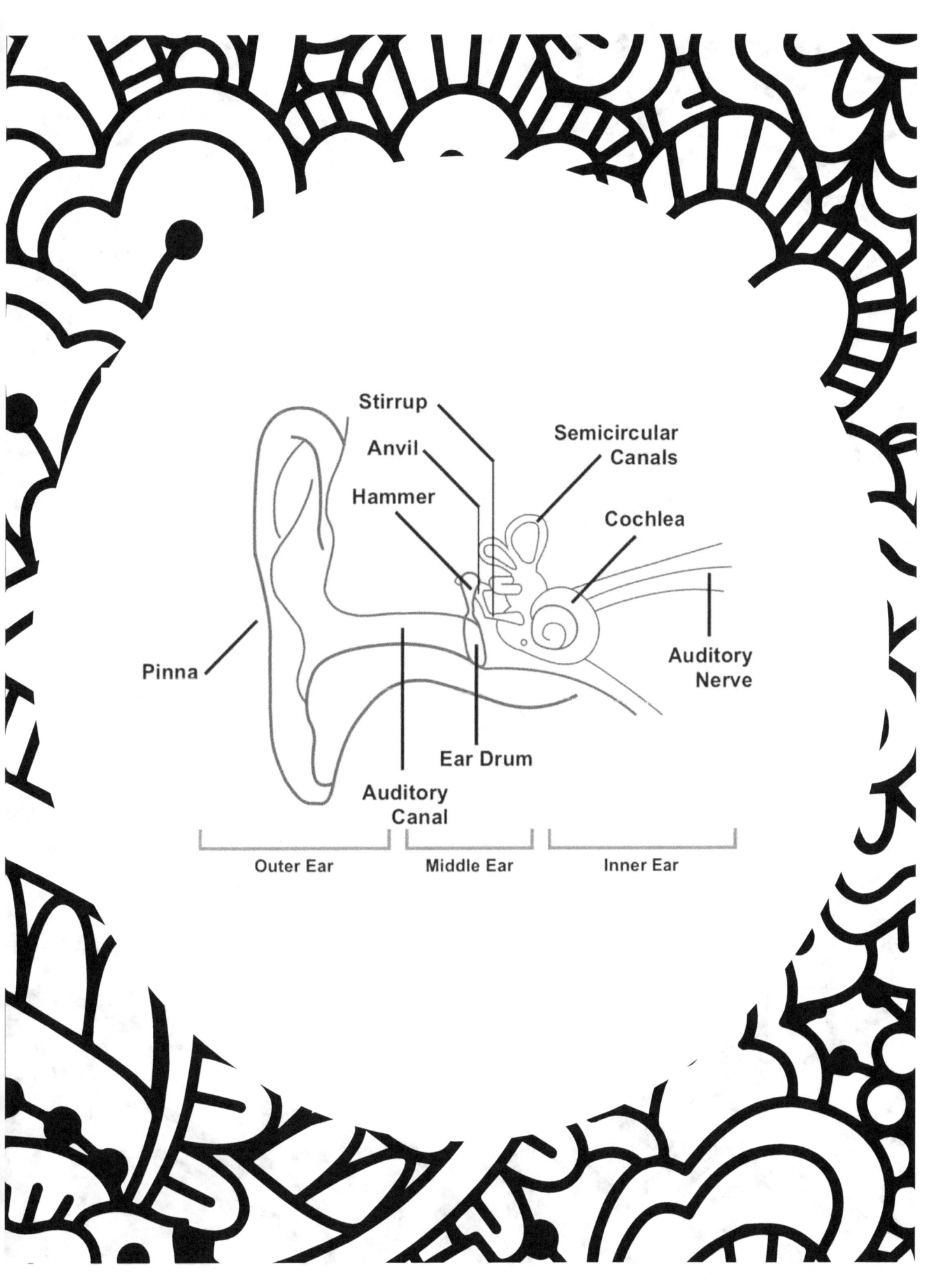

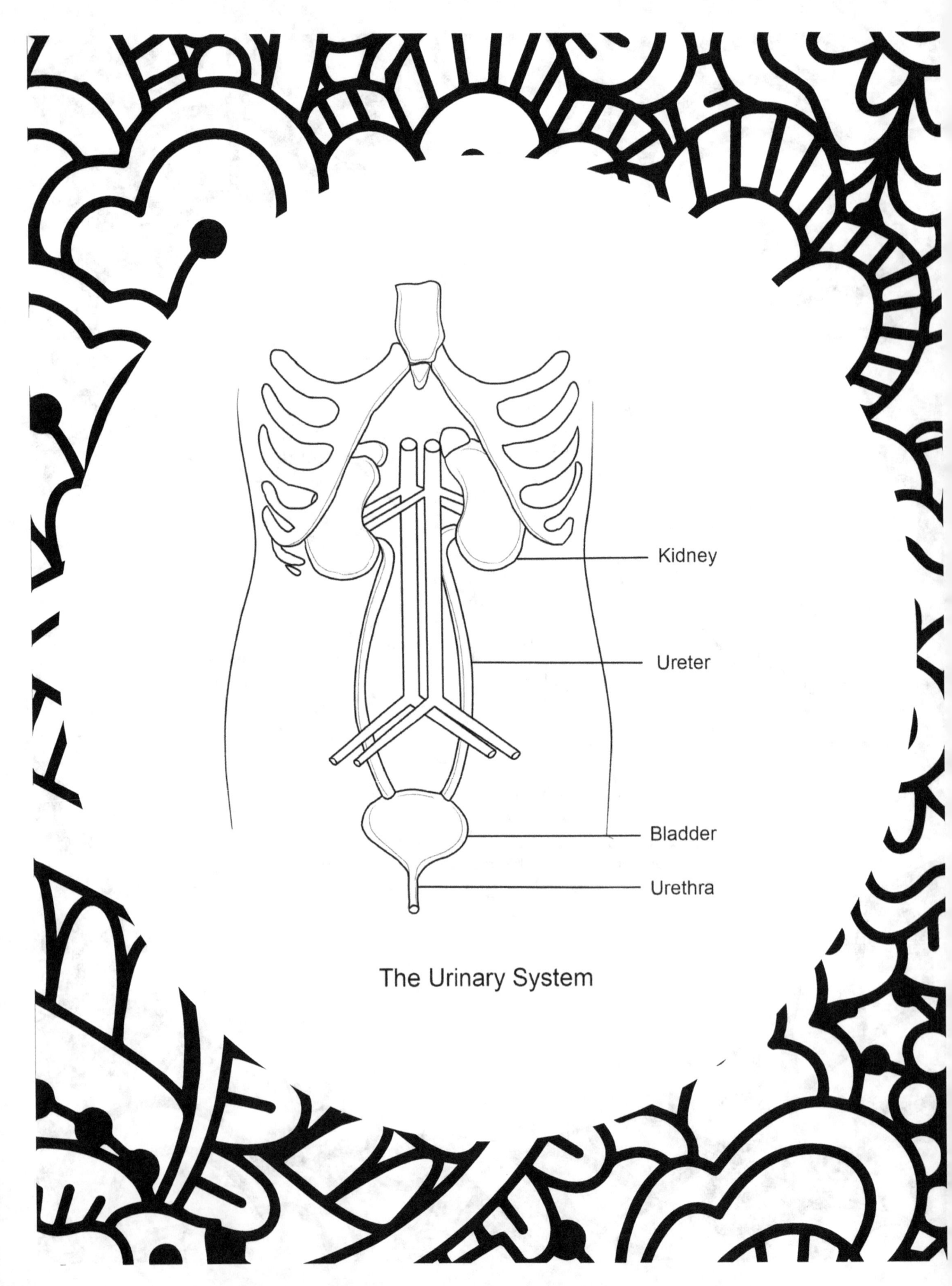

Kidney

Ureter

Bladder

Urethra

The Urinary System

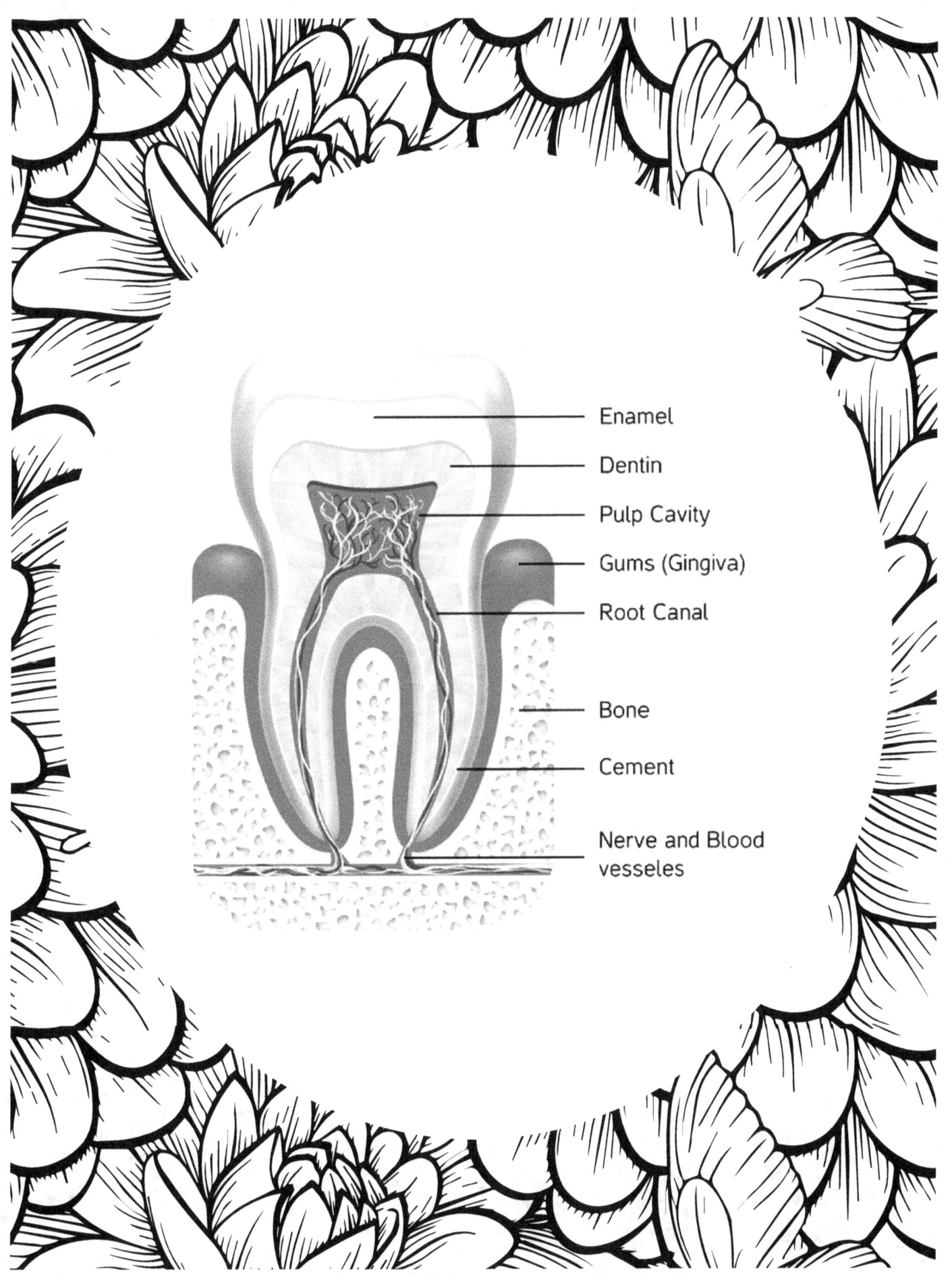

Enamel

Dentin

Pulp Cavity

Gums (Gingiva)

Root Canal

Bone

Cement

Nerve and Blood vesseles

HUMAN BRAIN -SIDE VIEW

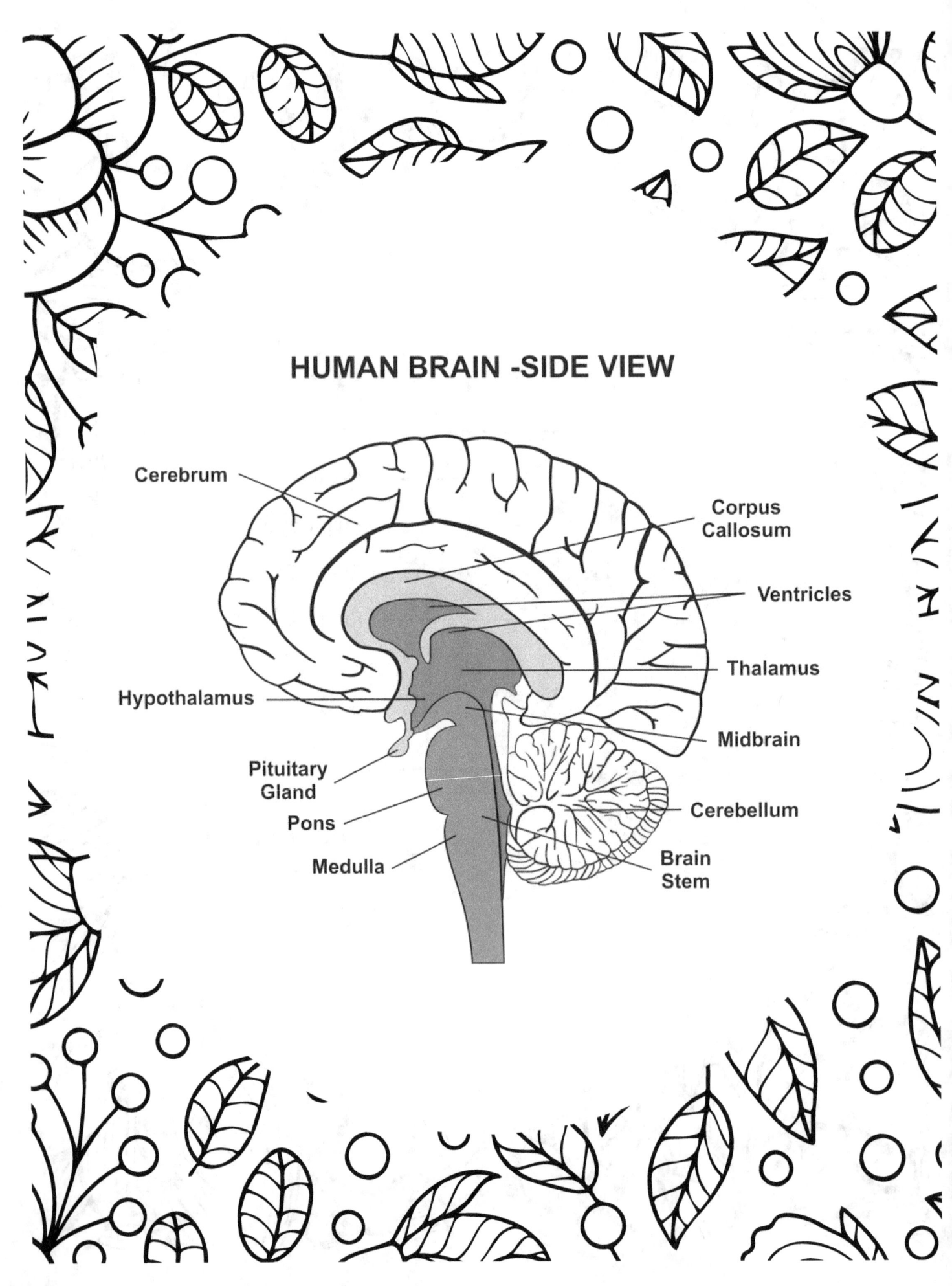

Cerebrum

Corpus Callosum

Ventricles

Thalamus

Hypothalamus

Midbrain

Pituitary Gland

Cerebellum

Pons

Medulla

Brain Stem

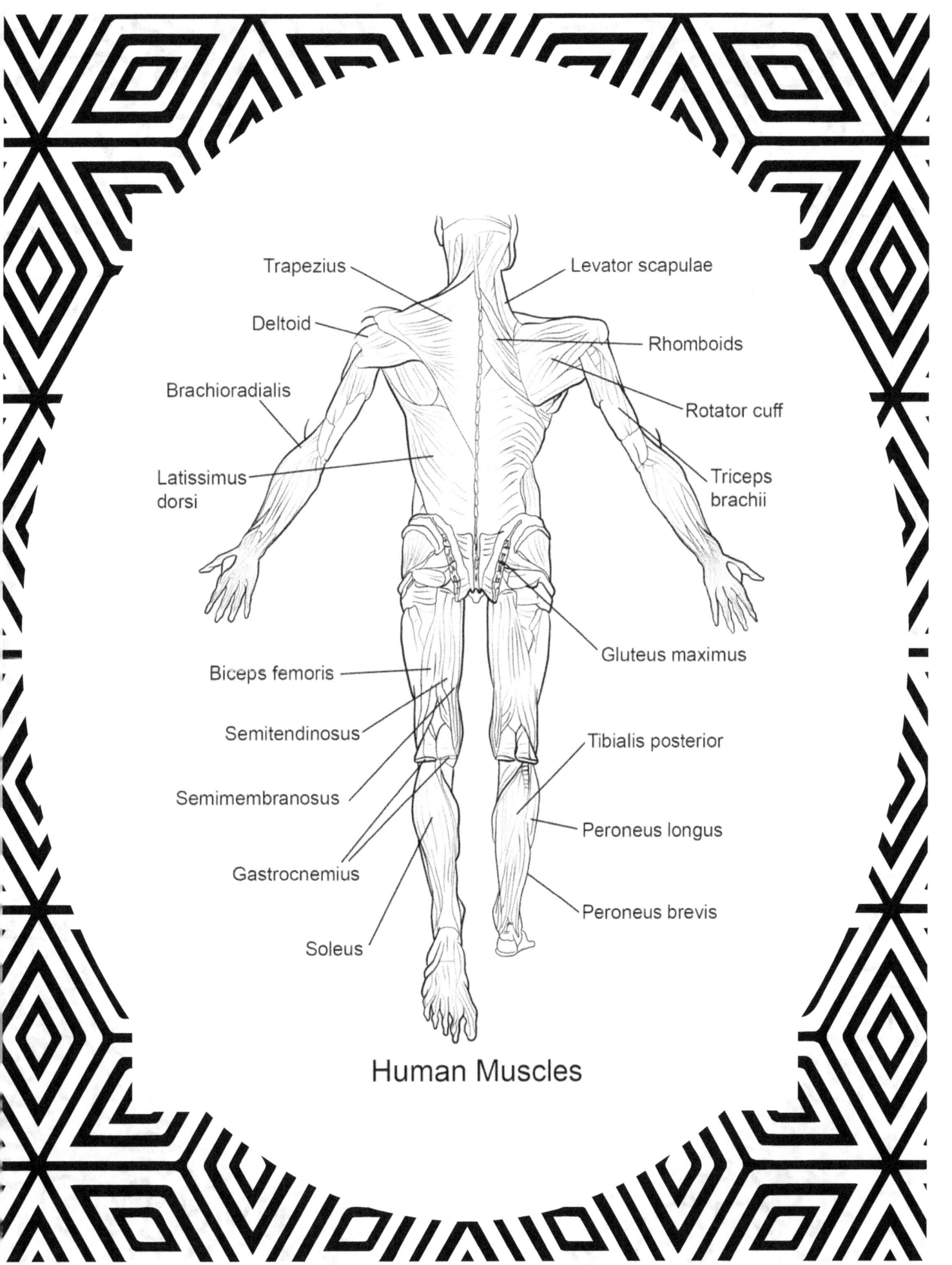

Human Muscles

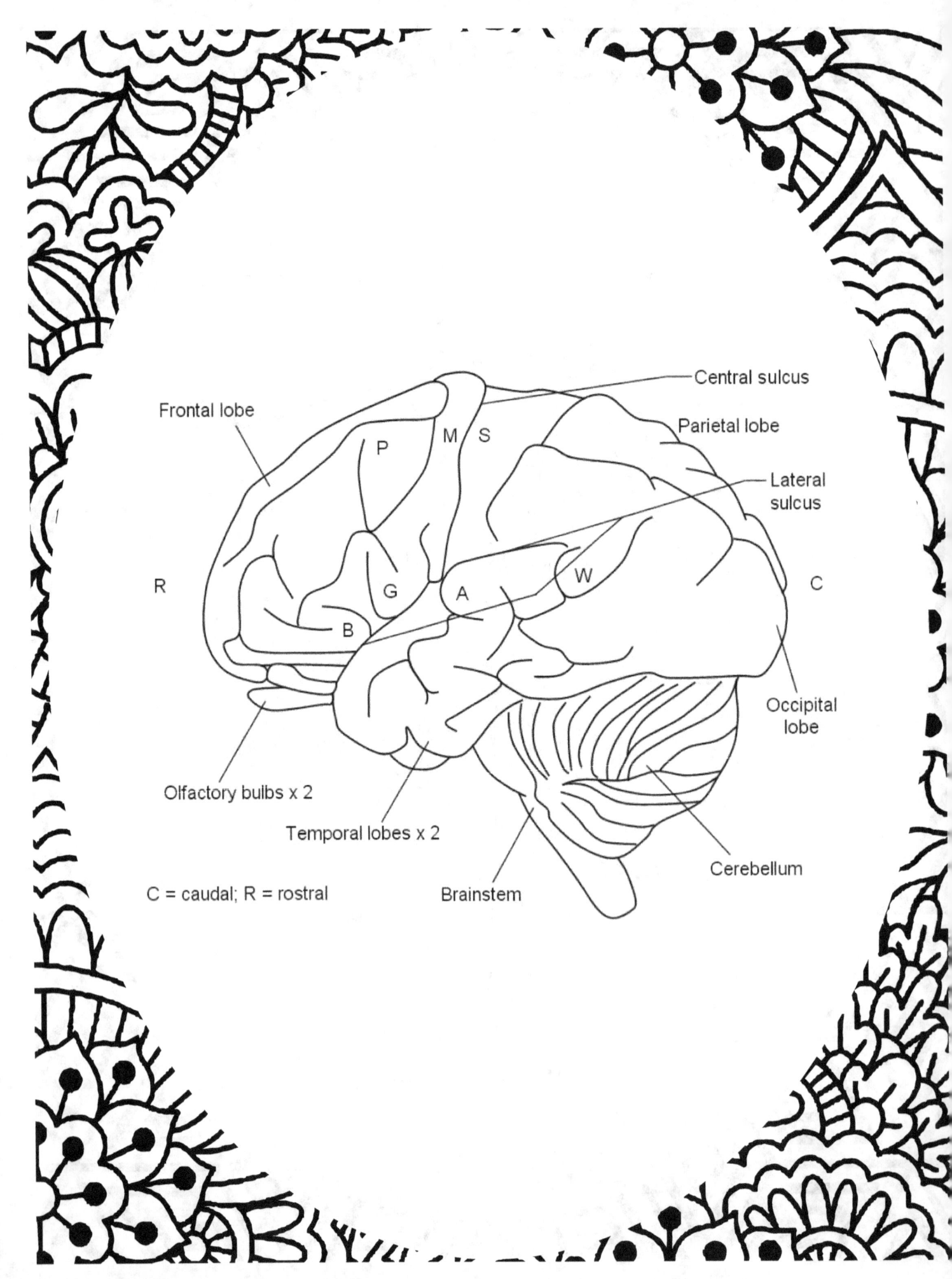

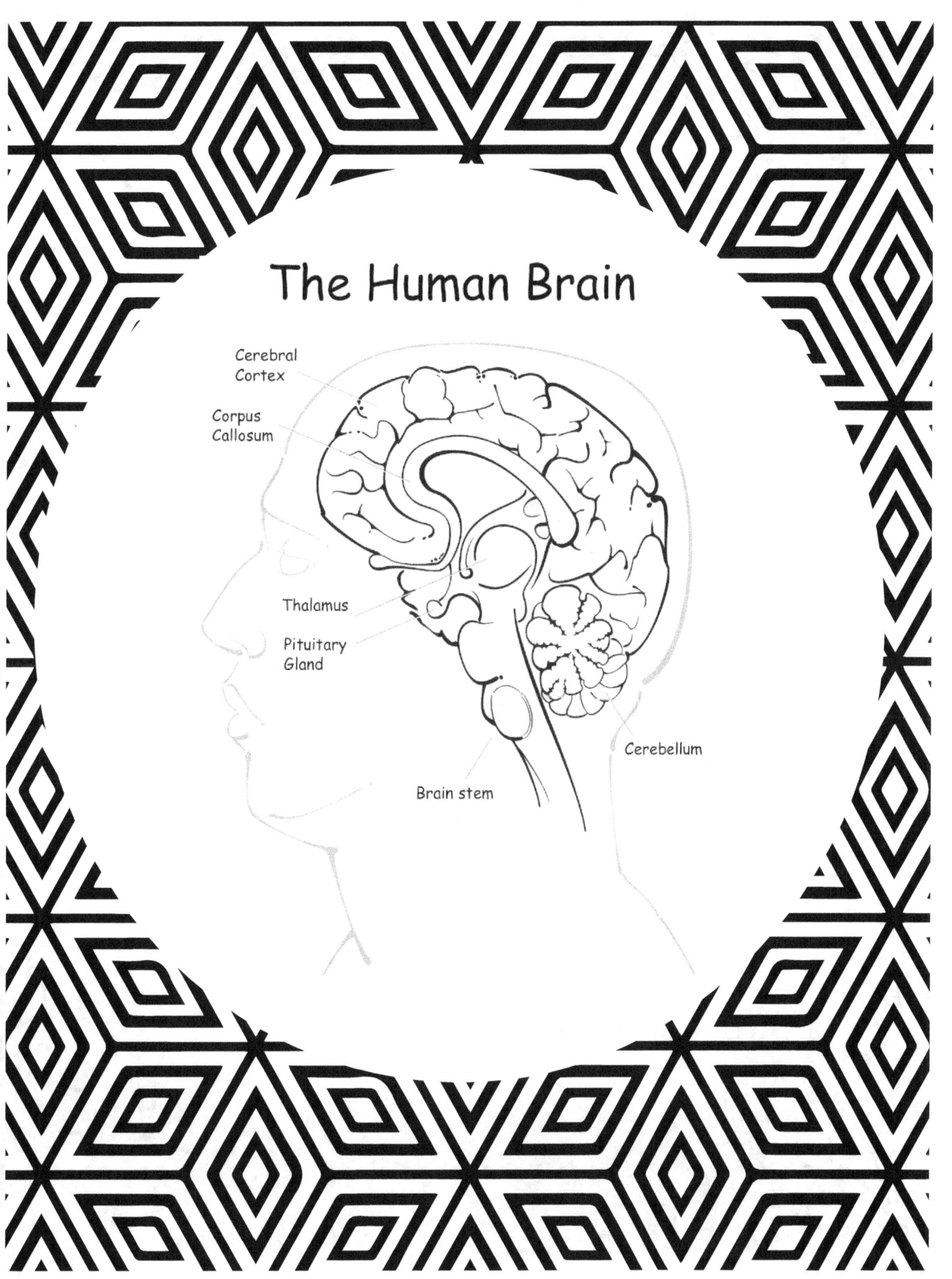

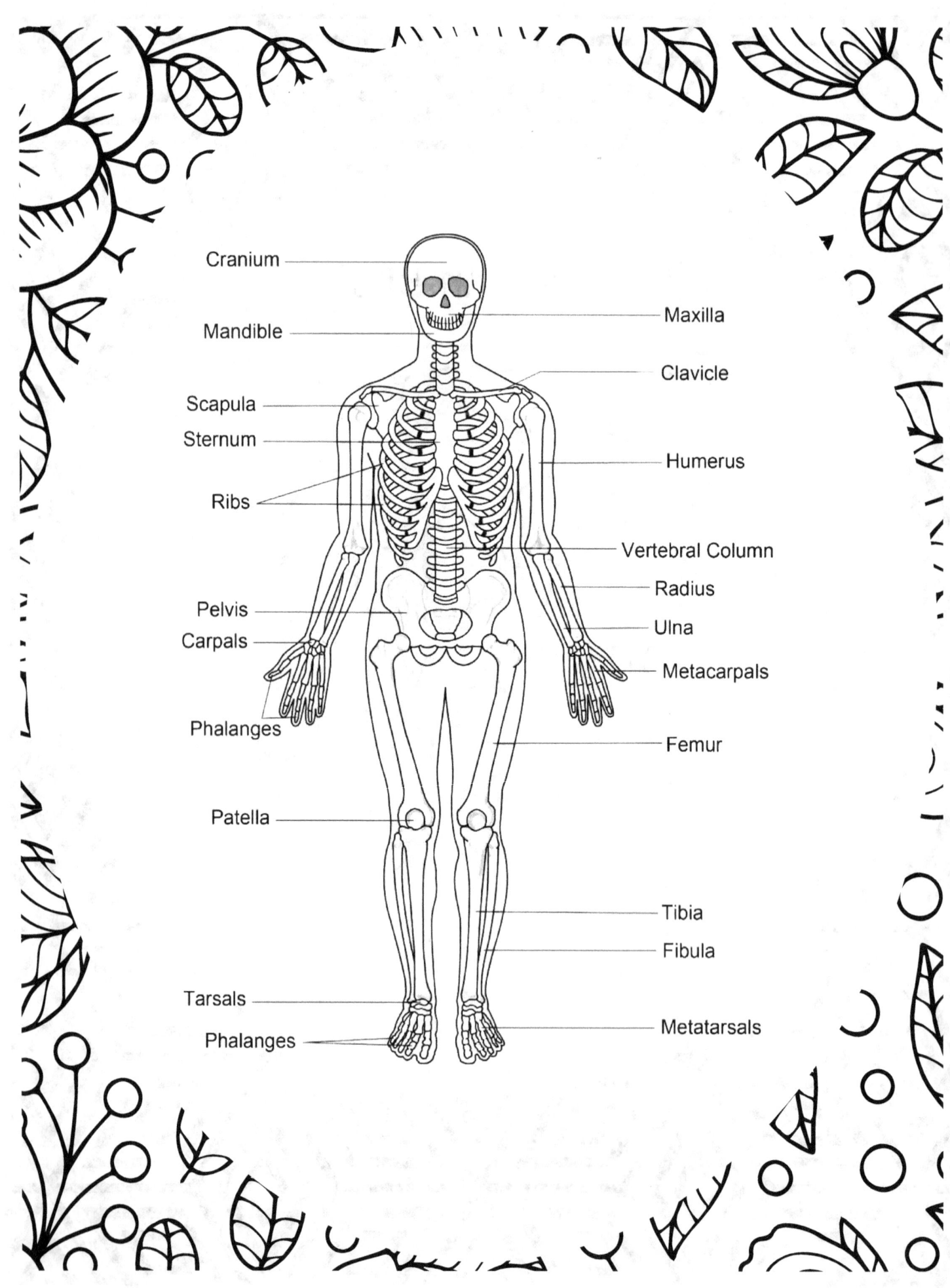

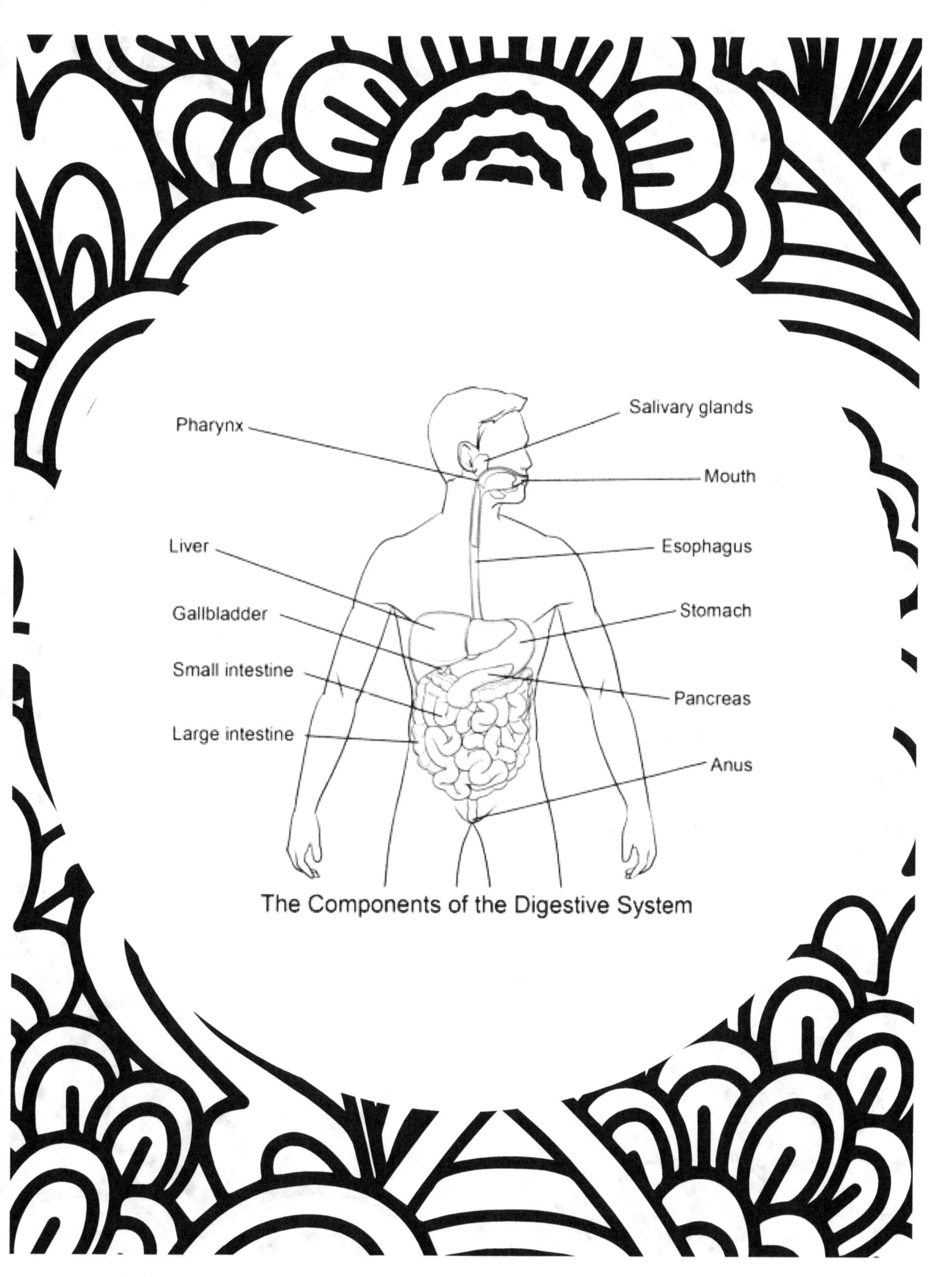

The Components of the Digestive System

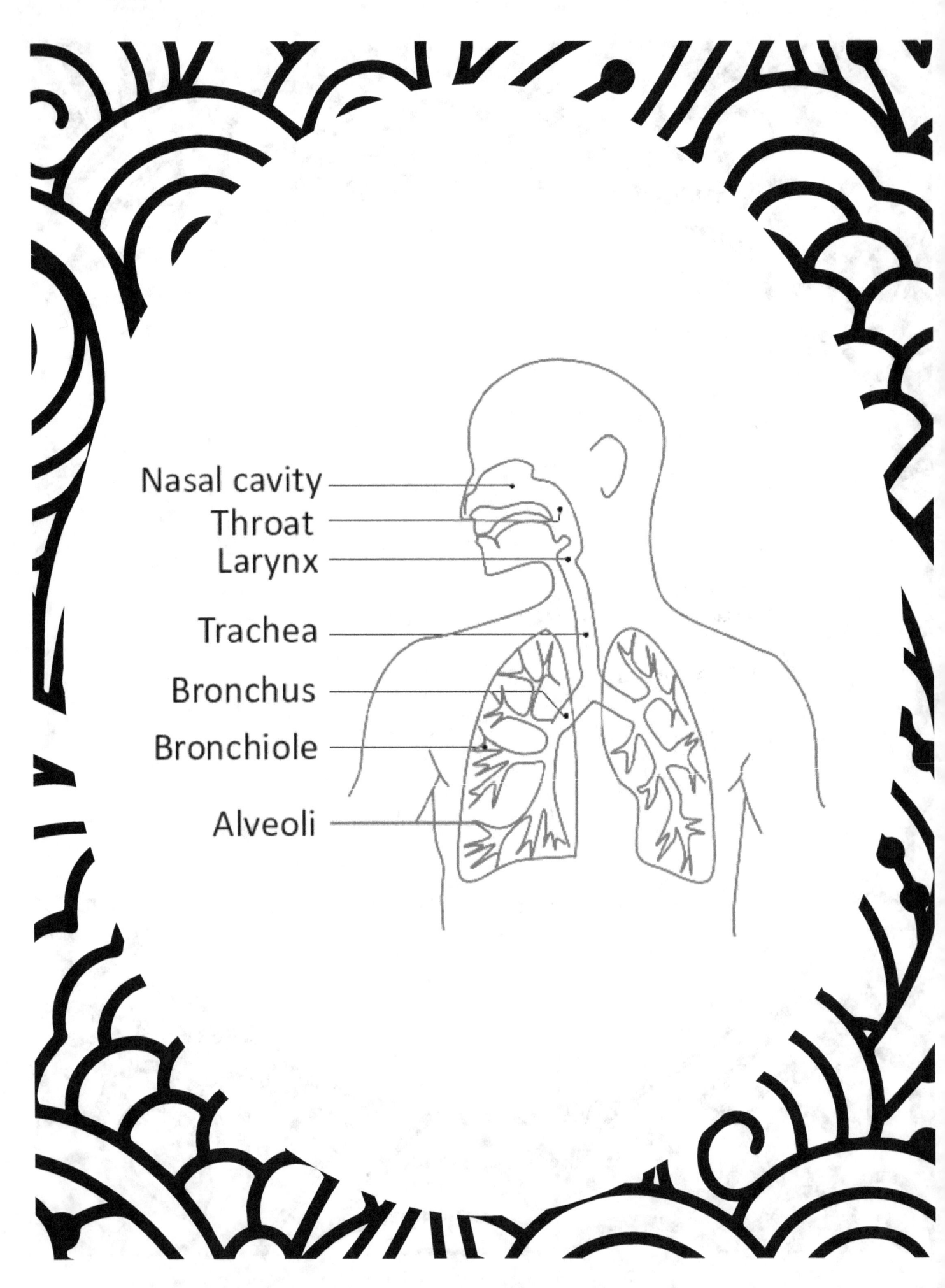

www.ingramcontent.com/pod-product-compliance
Lightning Source LLC
Chambersburg PA
CBHW081701220526

45466CB00009B/2842